2022
国际医学教育研究前沿报告

International Medical Education Research Fronts Report

闻德亮　李鸿鹤　著

科学出版社

北　京

内 容 简 介

《2022 国际医学教育研究前沿报告》是本系列丛书的第五册，也是重要的阶段性总结。因此，本报告通过文献计量学和文本挖掘技术，基于 Web of Science 数据库，全面梳理并揭示了 2021 年度全球医学教育的发展状态和前沿热点；回顾并比较了二十年来（2001—2020 年）全球医学教育的发展状态和研究热点；聚焦全球医学教育教学研究，分析教育教学板块的发展状态和前沿热点；构建医学教育研究领域专有的 ESI 机构统计排名；解析国际医学教育研究期刊，描绘其外部特征和发表兴趣取向，为医学教育研究者提供重要参考。同时，在本年度的研究前沿报告中，与时俱进地引入了重点研究议题"医学教育模式的实践与展望"进行专题介绍，以期能够帮助全球的医学教育研究者、工作者紧跟时代步伐，共促医学教育的长足发展。

本书可供国内外医学教育研究者、工作者参考使用。

图书在版编目（CIP）数据

2022 国际医学教育研究前沿报告/闻德亮，李鸿鹤著.—北京：科学出版社，2022.11

ISBN 978-7-03-073898-1

Ⅰ.①2… Ⅱ.①闻… ②李… Ⅲ.①医学教育－研究报告－世界－2022 Ⅳ.①R-4

中国版本图书馆 CIP 数据核字（2022）第 220518 号

责任编辑：王 颖/责任校对：宁辉彩
责任印制：李 彤/封面设计：陈 敬

科学出版社 出版
北京东黄城根北街 16 号
邮政编码：100717
http://www.sciencep.com
北京建宏印刷有限公司 印刷
科学出版社发行 各地新华书店经销
*
2022 年 11 月第 一 版 开本：720×1000 1/16
2023 年 1 月第二次印刷 印张：6
字数：138 000
定价：45.00 元
（如有印装质量问题，我社负责调换）

序

　　建设教育强国是中华民族伟大复兴的基础工程；人民健康是民族昌盛和国家富强的重要标志。因此，培养高水平医学卫生人才是全球高等医学教育机构的时代担当。随着全球化发展不断深入，全球医学教育事业和卫生健康事业都进入了一个新的历史发展阶段。如何实现更好的医学教育，要求全球的医学教育研究者、工作者紧跟医学教育脉搏，加强互相了解，及时更新先进的教育教学理念，与世界发展共频。

　　中国医科大学作为中国较早开展西医学学院式教育的高等学校，始终致力于为人类卫生健康事业发展做出积极贡献，在高等医学教育研究与改革方面积累了丰富的经验。中国医科大学国际医学教育研究院经过 30 余年的探索与发展，借鉴国际先进医学教育理念和经验，结合中国国情进行研究实践，取得了具有中国特色的医学教育改革和研究成果，并将成果推广应用。作为以"育人为本，国际视野，立足国情，服务社会"为使命的国际化医学教育研究机构，有责任也有义务向国家宏观决策层、专家学者和社会全面系统地报告国际医学教育研究的发展情况，对未来发展进行前瞻性的思考和展望。

　　为更好地融入并推动医学教育的理论研究和改革发展，我们迫切需要一部全球医学教育发展指南来指导中国的医学教育工作者从事医疗教育实践的教学与研究，"国际医学教育研究前沿报告"正是利用这一契机编写的一部具有前沿意义的医学教育发展指南，为国内外众多医学院校和专家学者提供了追踪全球医学教育整体态势和发展变化的机会。本研究报告的发布离不开科睿唯安团队的通力合作与科学出版社的大力支持。我们在编写过程中力争保证资料的全面性和准确性，并且参与该项目的专家学者们开展了一系列的研讨会、审稿会等，将撰写的每一个细节力争做到最好。如有疏漏之处，恳请各位同道和读者批评指正。

闻德亮

2022 年 10 月 10 日

前　言

医学教育是卫生健康事业发展的重要基石。党的十八大以来，我国医学教育蓬勃发展，为卫生健康事业输送了大批高素质医学人才。2022 年正值实施"十四五"规划的关键之年，也是我国构建新发展格局显现成效的一年，面对新冠肺炎疫情提出的持续挑战、实施健康中国战略的持续任务、世界医学发展的持续要求，迫切需要一部关于国内外医学教育的发展指南来帮助我国的医学教育工作者更好地从事医学教育实践的教学和研究，推进医学教育创新发展。"国际医学教育研究前沿报告"系列丛书的出版恰逢其时，是一部具有先进指导意义的医学教育发展指南。本系列丛书对医学教育领域整体态势及发展变化做出了综合概括描述，利用科学计量学技术揭示国际上医学教育研究的发展特征和研究前沿，进而把握国际医学教育的动态发展变化。

"国际医学教育研究前沿报告"系列丛书自 2018 年出版至今已走过 5 个春秋，内容不断地更新和丰富，与时俱进地引入了国际上的最新研究成果。今年，我们在延续原有内容板块和主导思想的基础上，兼顾过去与未来，回首过去与展望未来并行，针对 20 年来的国际医学教育文献，以 5 年为一个时间段，探讨其发展特征与研究热点的迭代变化。同时，针对医学教育教学研究的发展需求和广大读者的期待，在书中新增了另外两部分内容，旨在从多角度探索医学教育研究的发展脉络。两个新增的部分是：全球医学教育教学研究专题分析，以及国际上重点研究议题"医学教育模式的实践与展望"的专题介绍。

至此，《2022 国际医学教育研究前沿报告》已经涵盖了最新年度和 20 年来医学教育研究论文的外部特征描绘、热点和前沿研究主题内容挖掘和聚类分析、国际新兴和重点议题的专题介绍、国际医学教育教学研究专题分析、国际医学教育研究机构 ESI 排名和国际期刊统计分析等全面丰富的内容板块，旨在为国内外医学教育工作者提供完整的研究概况。本书通过揭示全球医学教育的研究现状和热点前沿，帮助全球的医学教育工作者紧跟国际医学教育整体发展态势，并对未来发展进行前瞻性的思考和展望，使得处于疫情防控常态化的医学教育变得有迹可循、有理可依。在未来的研究中，"国际医学教育研究前沿报告"也将贯彻落实习近平总书记关于教育的重要论述，坚持正确政治方向，紧跟新时代推进高等教育高质量发展，致力于全面提高医学生人才培养能力，为我国的医疗卫生和医学教育事业添砖加瓦。

最后感谢中国医科大学编者团队——曲波教授、崔雷教授、赵阳助理研究员，以及国际医学教育研究院的博、硕士研究生宋鑫智、江南、崔雪梅、辛春雨、李颖等的辛勤工作，我们坚信"国际医学教育研究前沿报告"系列丛书将对全球医学教育的改革发展大有裨益，在未来的发展中一定会越办越好！

闻德亮

2022 年 10 月 10 日

目　　录

2022 International Medical Education Research Fronts Report

2022 国际医学教育研究前沿报告

（中文部分）

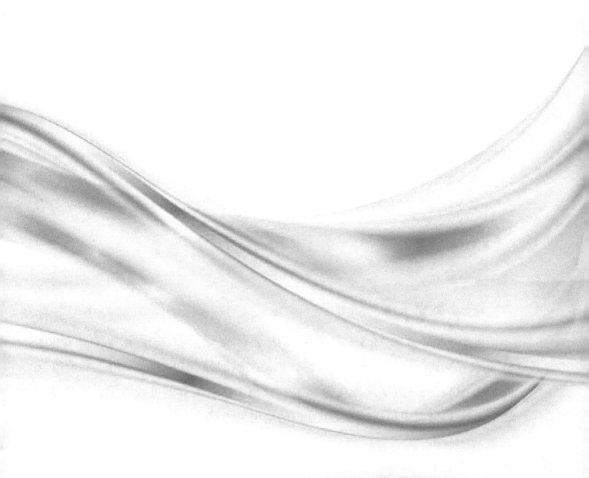

背　　景

　　医学教育的国际化进程逐步加快，形成了全球性的相互依存，这种趋势要求我们必须要加强互相了解，及时更新理念，掌握国际医学教育研究的现状和发展趋势，从而不断开拓医学教育研究与改革的新未来。2018—2021 年我们连续四年发布了国际医学教育研究系列前沿报告，获得了国内外医学教育界的强烈反响。2022 年是国际医学教育研究系列前沿报告发布的第五年，我们在延续原有内容板块的基础上，对 2001 年至 2020 年国际医学教育研究文献进行了概览与热点回顾，并进行了关于全球医学教育教学研究的专题探讨。我们希望通过这样一个平台，能够帮助全球的医学教育研究者、工作者紧跟时代步伐，把握国际医学教育的整体发展态势，对未来发展进行前瞻性的思考和展望。

目　　的

　　基于 Web of Science 和 PubMed 数据库：

　　（一）梳理并揭示 2021 年度全球医学教育研究热点和发展状态。

　　（二）回顾并比较 2001—2020 年全球医学教育研究热点和发展状态。

　　（三）聚焦全球医学教育教学研究，分析医学教育教学板块的研究热点和发展状态。

　　（四）构建医学教育研究领域 ESI 机构统计排名。

　　（五）描绘医学教育研究期刊外部特征和发表兴趣取向，为医学教育研究者提供重要参考。

方　　法

（一）数据采集

　　利用 PubMed 的 MeSH 主题词方法进行检索，收集标引为"Education, Medical"及其下位类主题词的文献，确定文献的独有 PMID 号，并与科睿唯安的 Web of Science 数据库（均为 SCIE 或 SSCI 收录文章）进行匹配，下载 Web of Science 数据库中包括参考文献在内的全记录题录。

（二）文献概览

在第一步数据集收集整理的基础上，基于 Web of Science 数据库文献题录的信息和分类，利用科学计量学软件 HistCite 及可视化分析工具 CiteSpace 对如下指标进行统计分析，包括：高发文量国家（地区）分布、高被引量国家（地区）分布、高发文量机构分布、高被引量机构分布、高发文量作者分布和高被引量作者分布。

（三）研究前沿

1. 高频主题词分布及聚类分析

在上述数据集收集整理的基础上，利用书目共现分析系统 BICOMB 对来源文献的 MeSH Terms 字段进行主要主题词提取，生成高频主题词列表。高频主题词聚类通过将生成的高频主题词词篇矩阵导入聚类工具 gCLUTO 实现。

2. 引文共被引聚类分析

引文共被引聚类是通过对共同出现在施引文献中的被引文献间关系的分析来反映被引文献间聚集程度的一种聚类方式。本研究基于书目共现分析系统 BICOMB 对纳入本次分析的文献集的引文进行抽取、排序并生成共被引矩阵，最终进行聚类分析。

结　　果

一、2021 年国际医学教育研究文献概览及研究前沿分析

检索策略：MeSH 主题词 "Education, Medical" + JCR 数据库中教育门类下 10 种医学教育期刊（*Academic Medicine / Medical Education / Medical Teacher / BMC Medical Education / Journal of Surgical Education / Advances in Health Sciences Education / Teaching and Learning in Medicine / Medical Education Online / Anatomical Sciences Education / Academic Psychiatry*）。

（一）文献概览

1. 国际医学教育论文 2021 年发文量及被引量的国家 / 地区分布（图 1）

序号	国家 / 地区	发文量	百分比*		序号	国家 / 地区	被引量	百分比*	平均被引量
1	美国	4026	45.53		1	美国	5247	43.63	1.30
2	英国	776	8.78		2	英国	1013	8.42	1.31
3	加拿大	630	7.12		3	加拿大	944	7.85	1.50
4	澳大利亚	286	3.23		4	荷兰	514	4.27	2.16
5	荷兰	238	2.69		5	澳大利亚	505	4.20	1.77
6	德国	229	2.59		6	中国	302	2.51	1.44
7	中国	210	2.37		7	德国	228	1.90	1.00
8	印度	143	1.62		8	爱尔兰	204	1.70	2.19
9	法国	127	1.44		9	意大利	199	1.65	1.67
10	意大利	119	1.35		10	印度	189	1.57	1.32
11	瑞士	103	1.16		11	法国	139	1.16	1.09
12	巴西	93	1.05		12	瑞士	130	1.08	1.26
13	爱尔兰	93	1.05		13	波兰	126	1.05	4.06
14	日本	83	0.94		14	沙特阿拉伯	125	1.04	1.89
15	新加坡	83	0.94		15	日本	122	1.01	1.47

图 1　国际医学教育论文 2021 年发文量及被引量的国家 / 地区分布

2. 国际医学教育论文 2021 年发文量及被引量的机构分布（图 2）

序号	机构	发文量	百分比*		序号	机构	被引量	百分比*	平均被引量
1	哈佛大学医学院	291	1.49		1	哈佛大学医学院	448	1.57	1.54
2	加州大学旧金山分校	222	1.14		2	加州大学旧金山分校	399	1.40	1.80
3	密歇根大学	204	1.04		3	密歇根大学	371	1.30	1.82
4	华盛顿大学	201	1.03		4	华盛顿大学	370	1.30	1.84
5	多伦多大学	194	0.99		5	多伦多大学	352	1.24	1.81
6	斯坦福大学	178	0.91		6	斯坦福大学	299	1.05	1.68
7	梅奥医学中心	155	0.79		7	宾夕法尼亚大学	285	1.00	1.91
8	宾夕法尼亚大学	149	0.76		8	梅奥医学中心	268	0.94	1.73
9	范德堡大学	135	0.69		9	马斯特里赫特大学	227	0.80	2.64
10	麻省总医院	126	0.64		10	北卡罗来纳大学	227	0.80	2.01
11	约翰斯·霍普金斯大学	124	0.63		11	范德堡大学	218	0.77	1.61
12	西北大学	116	0.59		12	麻省总医院	201	0.71	1.60
13	埃默里大学	113	0.58		13	西北大学	194	0.68	1.67
14	北卡罗来纳大学	113	0.58		14	不列颠哥伦比亚大学	172	0.60	1.83
15	俄亥俄州立大学	109	0.57		15	伊利诺伊大学	172	0.60	2.57

图 2　国际医学教育论文 2021 年发文量及被引量的机构分布

---

* 本书中百分比单位为 1%。

3. 国际医学教育论文 2021 年发文量及被引量的作者分布（图 3）

序号	高发文作者	所在机构	发文量
1	Hauer, Karen E.	加州大学旧金山分校	23
2	Park, Yoon Soo	哈佛大学医学院	23
3	Hammoud, Maya M.	密歇根大学	22
4	Schumacher, Daniel J.	辛辛那提大学	20
5	Santen, Sally A.	弗吉尼亚联邦大学	19
6	Ten Cate, Olle	乌得勒支大学医学中心	19
7	Drolet, Brain C.	范德堡大学	17
8	O'Sullivan, Patricia S.	加州大学旧金山分校	16
9	Teunissen, Pim W.	马斯特里赫特大学	16
10	Varpio, Lara	健康科学统一服务大学	15
11	Cleland, Jennifer	南洋理工大学	14
12	Driessen, Erik W.	马斯特里赫特大学	14
13	George, Brian C.	密歇根大学	14
14	Ross, Shelley	阿尔伯塔大学	13
15	Elkbuli, Adel	肯德尔地区医疗中心	13

序号	高被引作者	所在机构	被引量	平均被引量
1	Varpio, Lara	健康科学统一服务大学	72	4.80
2	Ten Cate, Olle	乌得勒支大学医学中心	63	3.32
3	Asaad, Malke	得克萨斯大学安德森癌症中心	61	5.55
4	Dumont, Aaron S.	杜兰大学	60	15
5	Teunissen, Pim W.	马斯特里赫特大学	59	3.69
6	Aziz, Hassan	南加州大学	57	28.50
7	Iwanaga, Joe	杜兰大学	57	28.50
8	Sullivan, Maura E.	南加州大学	57	19.00
9	Tubbs, R. Shane	杜兰大学	57	14.25
10	Genyk, Yuri	南加州大学	56	56
11	Remulla, Daphne	南加州大学	56	56
12	Sheikh, Mohd Raashid	南加州大学	56	56
13	Sher, Linda	南加州大学	56	56
14	James, Tayler	南加州大学	56	56
15	Loukas, Marios	奥尔什丁瓦尔米亚玛祖里大学	54	54

图 3　国际医学教育论文 2021 年发文量及被引量的作者分布

注：作者分布统计对所有发文作者的贡献同等对待，不区分第一作者、通讯作者与合著作者。

（二）研究前沿

1. 国际医学教育论文 2021 年高频主题词分布（图 4）

序号	主题词	频次	百分比	序号	主题词	频次	百分比
1	Internship and Residency	3220	13.39	21	Surgery, Plastic	161	0.67
2	Students, Medical	1547	6.43	22	Psychiatry	149	0.62
3	COVID-19	1267	5.27	23	Schools, Medical	139	0.58
4	Education, Medical	1226	5.10	24	Education, Medical, Continuing	133	0.55
5	Education, Medical, Undergraduate	947	3.94	25	Pediatrics	120	0.50
6	Education, Medical, Graduate	533	2.22	26	Learning	120	0.50
7	Clinical Competence	432	1.80	27	Orthopedics	113	0.47
8	Physicians	387	1.61	28	Emergency Medicine	111	0.46
9	General Surgery	352	1.46	29	Dermatology	110	0.46
10	Education, Distance	295	1.23	30	Teaching Rounds	109	0.45
11	Curriculum	292	1.21	31	Ophthalmology	109	0.45
12	Surgeons	268	1.11	32	Faculty, Medical	105	0.44
13	Educational Measurement	233	0.97	33	Obstetrics	100	0.42
14	Simulation Training	201	0.84	34	Gynecology	100	0.42
15	Anatomy	183	0.76	35	Medicine	100	0.42
16	Radiology	174	0.72	36	Otolaryngology	100	0.42
17	Pandemics	173	0.72	37	Urology	99	0.41
18	Fellowships and Scholarships	165	0.69	38	Biomedical Research	98	0.41
19	Clinical Clerkship	164	0.68	39	Personnel Selection	95	0.40
20	Burnout, Professional	163	0.68	40	Neurosurgery	95	0.40

图 4　国际医学教育论文 2021 年高频主题词分布

2. 国际医学教育论文 2021 年高频主题词聚类（图 5）

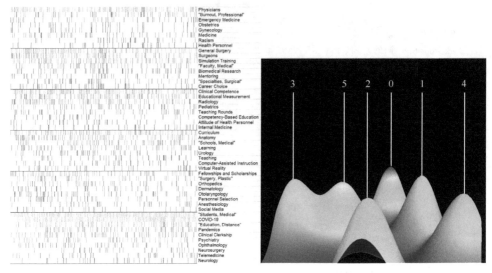

图 5　国际医学教育论文 2021 年高频主题词聚类

注：右图中数字表示高频主题词聚类所形成的主题类别。

通过高频主题词聚类分析，2021 年国际医学教育研究主题涵盖以下 6 个主要方面：

（1）医务人员执业环境及影响因素研究。

（2）医学院校教师职业发展研究。

（3）以临床胜任力为导向的教学与评价研究。

（4）数字化信息技术在医学教学中的应用。

（5）在新冠肺炎疫情影响下，社交媒体在卫生人力资源配置中发挥的作用。

（6）在新冠肺炎疫情影响下，医学教学模式和方法改革研究。

专题介绍：医学教育模式的实践与展望

近年来，全球医学教育正经历着关键性的变革，2010 年掀起的第三代医学教育改革浪潮以及当下新冠肺炎疫情的流行促使人们对医学教育进行再反思。在这样的历史时期中，医学教育模式迎来了新一轮的全球变革，相关研究也逐步展开。

1. 医学教育模式种类

医学教育模式是特定时代背景、特定的学习者、学习内容和学习环境相结合的产物，包含教育目标、教育内容、人才培养路径等多方面内容，会随着医学的发展、医学模式的转型发生不断的演化。在整个发展进程中，医学教育模式经历了三次重要的变革与升级，分别是经验医学教育模式、科学医学教育模式和人本医学教育模式（图6）。其中，科学医学教育模式是对18世纪至20世纪末期间的医学教育模式的统称，可以划分为基于学科的教育模式和基于问题的教育模式两个发展阶段。

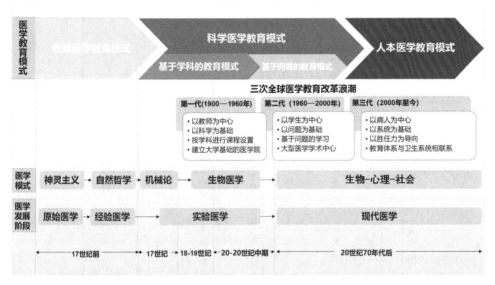

图6　医学教育模式变迁示意图

医学教育模式的革新离不开当时特定的时代背景、人们对医学认知的突破，以及社会需求的转变。特定的医学发展阶段决定了当时的医学模式，医学模式结合特定时代的学习者、学习内容和学习环境，共同决定了当下的医学教育模式。如图6所示，原始医学和经验医学背景下形成的神灵主义和自然哲学医学模式，决定了当时的经验医学教育模式。在进入实验医学阶段也开启了科学医学教育模式的时代，在这个时期也经历了第一代和第二代的医学教育改革，尤其是第二代全球医学教育改革是基于学科和基于问题的医学教育模式的分水岭。尽管在20世纪70年代，逐渐进入了现代医学发展阶段，开启了"生物-心理-社会"医学模式，但是人本医学教育模式是随着第三代以岗位胜任力为导向的全球医学教育改革拉开序幕，且在未来将持续很长一段时间并不断地成熟和完善。

2. 医学教育模式实践

（1）医学教育模式的各国实践

从医学萌芽发展至今，在不同的医学教育模式下，不同的国家和学校成为各个时期医学教育模式的先锋代表。表1从各个国家在不同医学教育模式下开展医学教育的医学人才培养目标、路径、课程模式、教学方法、学习理论等方面进行了总结。

表 1　医学教育模式的各国实践

医学教育模式	时期	代表性国家和学校	教育目标	培养路径	课程模式	教学方法
经验医学教育模式	1900 年以前	意大利、萨勒诺医学院 中国	巫医；传教士；大夫	师徒制，学校式	师带徒；权威医学著作、宗教和哲学知识	口耳相授 实践教学
科学医学教育模式　基于学科的医学教育模式	1900—1960 年	美国、约翰斯·霍普金斯大学医学院 德国、夏瑞蒂医科大学 日本、东京大学医学部	适用型专科人才	美国 3 年制转变为 2+2 年制，又转变为 5 年制； 德国：2+1 年制； 日本：3+3 年制转变为 3+4 年制	经典医学课程模式：以学科为中心的基础-临床课程体系	封闭式教学，灌输式教学方法；床边教学
基于问题的医学教育模式	1960—2000 年	加拿大、麦克马斯特大学医学院 英国、邓迪大学医学院 日本、东京医科大学	综合发展型人才	加拿大和美国：4+4 年制（其中第一个 4 年为大学教育本科阶段，第二个 4 年为大学教育后的临床医学培养阶段）； 英国：7 年制； 日本：2+4+1 年制	整合课程	基于问题学习 PBL；标准化病人
人本医学教育模式	2000 年至今	美国、哈佛大学医学院 英国、牛津大学医学院	具有胜任力的卓越学人才	美国：4+4 年制（同上）； 英国：6 年制	以胜任力为导向，课程之间的横向整合和课程各阶段之间的纵向整合	多元化的教学方法，如基于案例的合作式学习

（2）我国的医学教育模式探索

在我国医学发展的悠久历史中，医学教育为推动医学学科的发展起到了关键作用，医学教育模式随着政治经济社会的发展几经变革。从以中医为主体到西医萌芽，在我国不同历史发展时期力求探索立足我国国情的医学教育模式，并取得了辉煌成就。

在经验医学教育模式时期，中国医学教育课程随社会背景变化几经变动，但均以中医经典为基础。中医医学教育经历了萌芽、发展、顶峰各个阶段。中国共产党成立后，许多革命根据地积极创建医学院校，学习苏联模式，大力发展医学教育。中国共产党领导的高等医学教育与国情的发展紧密联系在一起，形成了相对独立而完整的医学教育体系，为新中国医学教育的建立与发展奠定了基础。

新中国成立以后，党和人民政府制定我国教育方针和卫生与健康工作指导方针，明确了医学教育事业的教育、卫生等部门按照发展方向和任务，逐步形成我国特有的高等医学教育体系，正式步入科学医学教育模式。从 2011 年的全国医学教育改革工作会议以来，我国经历了一系列医学教育培养体系、机制体制等方面的深刻变革，为人本医学教育模式发展打下了坚实基础。

我国的医学教育资源丰富，医学教育规模居于世界前列，但从社会需求角度来看，我国仍存在较大的拔尖创新型医学人才缺口，医学教育资源仍然相对短缺；基层医生的需求空间须继续进一步释放，公共卫生管理体制机制需要深化改革。在这样的背景下，我国亟须探索出适合于我国现阶段需求的人本主义教育模式的实践道路。

人类历史的发展和社会的进步，决定了医学教育模式的诞生和演变。新时代以来，我国正处在医学教育模式转型的关键时期，通过人才培养目标的新要求、新的培养体系的建设，以及多学科的深度融合，正努力优化医学教育和医疗卫生体系供需关系，以新的医学教育模式促进医学教育的改革创新。

推荐阅读

[1] 闻德亮，丁宁. 中国共产党领导高等医学教育的发展历程、辉煌成就与经验启示 [J]. 中国高教研究，2021, (8): 17-25.

[2] 赵同领，曹云飞，柳亮，等. 医学教育模式的演变及其动因 [J]. 卫生职业教育，2011, 29(21): 5-7.

[3] 金中杰. 论医学模式的演变与医学教育课程的设置 [J]. 卫生职业教育，2003, 21(12): 6-9.

[4] 胡建鹏，翟双庆，王键. 中医学理论体系的形成与发展 [J]. 中医药临床杂志，2015, 27(8): 1051-1054.

[5] 高爱国. 新时期中国医学教育改革发展的解析与思路 [D]. 第四军医大学，2001.

[6] 郭永松. 医学教育模式初探 [J]. 医学教育，1989, 70(4): 1-3.

[7] 孙宝志. 世界医学课程模式改革百年历程与借鉴 [J]. 中华医学教育杂志，2012, 32(1): 1-7.

[8] Frenk J, Chen L, Bhutta Z A, et al. Health professionals for a new century: transforming education to strengthen health systems in an interdependent world[J]. Lancet, 2010, 376(9756): 1923-1958.

[9] Wijnen-Meijer M, Burdick W, Alofs L, et al. Stages and transitions in medical education around the world: Clarifying structures and terminology[J]. Medical Teacher, 2013, 35(4): 7.

[10] 李曼丽，丁若曦，张羽，等. 从认知科学到学习科学：过去、现状与未来 [J]. 清华大学教育研究，2018, 39(4): 29-39.

二、2001—2020 年国际医学教育研究文献概览及研究热点回顾

检索策略：MeSH 主题词 "Education, Medical" + JCR 数据库中教育门类下 10 种医学教育期刊（*Academic Medicine / Medical Education / Medical Teacher / BMC Medical Education / Journal of Surgical Education / Advances in Health Sciences Education / Teaching and Learning in Medicine / Medical Education Online / Anatomical Sciences Education / Academic Psychiatry*）。

统计年限：2001 年 1 月 1 日至 2020 年 12 月 31 日。

文献类型：限定为 Article。

（一）文献概览

1.国际医学教育论文 2001—2005 年发文量及被引量的国家 / 地区分布（图 7 ）

序号	国家 / 地区	发文量	百分比	序号	国家 / 地区	被引量	百分比	平均被引量
1	美国	4131	51.38	1	美国	142 730	52.88	34.55
2	英国	1177	14.64	2	英国	41 934	15.54	35.63
3	加拿大	674	8.38	3	加拿大	28 412	10.53	42.15
4	澳大利亚	332	4.13	4	荷兰	10 941	4.05	50.42
5	荷兰	217	2.70	5	澳大利亚	9266	3.43	27.91
6	德国	203	2.52	6	德国	3836	1.42	18.90
7	法国	96	1.19	7	以色列	2523	0.93	35.04
8	意大利	76	0.95	8	瑞典	2392	0.89	39.21
9	以色列	72	0.90	9	丹麦	2197	0.81	46.74
10	新西兰	62	0.77	10	新西兰	2064	0.76	33.29
11	瑞典	61	0.76	11	瑞士	1847	0.68	30.78
12	瑞士	60	0.75	12	意大利	1764	0.65	23.21
13	中国	58	0.72	13	巴西	1576	0.58	32.83
14	土耳其	54	0.67	14	比利时	1533	0.57	41.43
15	西班牙	53	0.66	15	挪威	1519	0.56	39.97

图 7　国际医学教育论文 2001—2005 年发文量及被引量的国家 / 地区分布

2.国际医学教育论文 2006—2010 年发文量及被引量的国家 / 地区分布（图 8 ）

序号	国家 / 地区	发文量	百分比	序号	国家 / 地区	被引量	百分比	平均被引量
1	美国	6159	44.67	1	美国	188 898	46.70	30.67
2	英国	1476	10.71	2	加拿大	44 086	10.90	39.43
3	加拿大	1118	8.11	3	英国	42 792	10.58	28.99
4	澳大利亚	571	4.14	4	荷兰	18 580	4.59	41.75
5	德国	520	3.77	5	澳大利亚	15 553	3.84	27.24
6	荷兰	445	3.23	6	德国	11 150	2.76	21.44
7	法国	207	1.50	7	意大利	4990	1.23	29.70
8	中国	170	1.23	8	法国	4591	1.13	22.18
9	意大利	168	1.22	9	西班牙	4118	1.02	25.74
10	西班牙	160	1.16	10	瑞典	4060	1.00	32.74
11	日本	136	0.99	11	瑞士	4012	0.99	30.63
12	巴西	131	0.95	12	日本	3812	0.94	28.03
13	瑞士	131	0.95	13	中国	3518	0.87	20.69
14	瑞典	124	0.90	14	丹麦	2994	0.74	35.64
15	以色列	97	0.71	15	比利时	2812	0.70	30.24

图 8　国际医学教育论文 2006—2010 年发文量及被引量的国家 / 地区分布

3. 国际医学教育论文 2011—2015 年发文量及被引量的国家 / 地区分布（图 9 ）

序号	国家 / 地区	发文量	百分比	序号	国家 / 地区	被引量	百分比	平均被引量
1	美国	7935	42.41	1	美国	174 489	42.24	21.99
2	加拿大	1724	9.21	2	加拿大	44 501	10.77	25.81
3	英国	1683	9.00	3	英国	44 017	10.65	26.15
4	澳大利亚	869	4.64	4	荷兰	21 253	5.14	29.85
5	德国	718	3.84	5	澳大利亚	18 894	4.57	21.74
6	荷兰	712	3.81	6	德国	12 488	3.02	17.39
7	中国	308	1.65	7	法国	5814	1.41	19.32
8	法国	301	1.61	8	瑞士	5780	1.40	26.15
9	瑞士	221	1.18	9	意大利	5619	1.36	26.50
10	意大利	212	1.13	10	比利时	4935	1.19	31.43
11	西班牙	197	1.13	11	中国	4725	1.14	15.34
12	巴西	188	1.05	12	丹麦	4269	1.03	25.11
13	日本	180	1.00	13	西班牙	3700	0.90	18.78
14	沙特阿拉伯	173	0.94	14	瑞典	3622	0.88	21.56
15	丹麦	170	0.91	15	巴西	3287	0.80	17.48

图 9　国际医学教育论文 2011—2015 年发文量及被引量的国家 / 地区分布

4. 国际医学教育论文 2016—2020 年发文量及被引量的国家 / 地区分布（图 10）

序号	国家 / 地区	发文量	百分比	序号	国家 / 地区	被引量	百分比	平均被引量
1	美国	9884	41.81	1	美国	94 268	41.83	9.54
2	加拿大	2029	8.58	2	加拿大	22 249	9.87	10.97
3	英国	1653	6.99	3	英国	16 613	7.37	10.05
4	澳大利亚	1096	4.64	4	澳大利亚	11 208	4.97	10.23
5	荷兰	921	3.90	5	荷兰	10 606	4.71	11.52
6	德国	882	3.73	6	德国	7711	3.42	8.74
7	中国	556	2.35	7	中国	4747	2.11	8.54
8	法国	403	1.70	8	意大利	3490	1.55	11.71
9	意大利	298	1.26	9	法国	3058	1.36	7.59
10	西班牙	296	1.25	10	西班牙	2705	1.20	9.14
11	瑞士	290	1.23	11	瑞士	2699	1.20	9.31
12	巴西	279	1.18	12	丹麦	2454	1.09	11.47
13	日本	259	1.10	13	爱尔兰	2317	1.03	10.21
14	印度	241	1.02	14	瑞典	2187	0.97	10.94
15	爱尔兰	227	0.96	15	比利时	2169	0.96	13.64

图 10　国际医学教育论文 2016—2020 年发文量及被引量的国家 / 地区分布

5. 国际医学教育论文 2001—2020 年发文量及被引量的国家 / 地区分布排名分析（图 11）

序号	国家 / 地区	发文量排名				序号	国家 / 地区	被引量排名			
		2001—2005	2006—2010	2011—2015	2016—2020			2001—2005	2006—2010	2011—2015	2016—2020
1	美国	1	1	1	1	1	美国	1	1	1	1
2	加拿大	3	3	2	2	2	加拿大	3	2	2	2
3	英国	2	2	3	3	3	英国	2	3	3	3
4	澳大利亚	4	4	4	4	4	澳大利亚	5	5	5	4
5	荷兰	5	6	6	5	5	荷兰	7	4	4	5
6	德国	6	5	5	6	6	德国	6	6	6	6
7	中国	13	8	7	7	7	中国	20	13	11	7
8	法国	7	7	8	8	8	意大利	12	7	7	8
9	意大利	9	9	10	9	9	法国	16	8	9	9
10	西班牙	15	10	11	10	10	西班牙	18	9	13	10
11	瑞士	12	12	9	11	11	瑞士	11	11	8	11
12	巴西	16	12	12	12	12	丹麦	9	14	12	12
13	日本	22	11	13	13	13	爱尔兰	21	16	17	13
14	印度	26	20	19	14	14	瑞典	8	12	14	14
15	爱尔兰	25	19	17	15	15	比利时	14	15	10	15

图 11　国际医学教育论文 2001—2020 年发文量及被引量的国家 / 地区分布排名分析

6. 国际医学教育论文 2001—2005 年发文量及被引量的机构分布（图 12）

序号	机构	发文量	百分比	序号	机构	被引量	百分比	平均被引量
1	多伦多大学	213	1.46	1	哈佛大学	11 670	2.24	56.38
2	哈佛大学	207	1.42	2	华盛顿大学	9772	1.88	51.43
3	得克萨斯大学	199	1.37	3	多伦多大学	9084	1.75	42.65
4	华盛顿大学	190	1.30	4	得克萨斯大学	6439	1.24	32.36
5	加州大学旧金山分校	156	1.07	5	耶鲁大学	6174	1.19	62.36
6	密歇根大学	127	0.87	6	加州大学旧金山分校	6130	1.18	39.29
7	宾夕法尼亚大学	105	0.72	7	西北大学	5454	1.05	65.71
8	匹兹堡大学	101	0.69	8	宾夕法尼亚大学	5253	1.01	50.03
9	耶鲁大学	99	0.68	9	密歇根大学	5073	0.97	39.94
10	北卡罗来纳大学	91	0.62	10	麦克马斯特大学	5063	0.97	61.74
11	加州大学洛杉矶分校	90	0.62	11	杜克大学	4694	0.90	67.06
12	约翰斯·霍普金斯大学	87	0.60	12	布莱根妇女医院	4448	0.85	98.84
13	西北大学	83	0.57	13	约翰斯·霍普金斯大学	3654	0.70	42.00
14	麦克马斯特大学	82	0.56	14	马斯特里赫特大学	3634	0.70	66.07
15	伊利诺伊大学	81	0.56	15	埃默里大学	3527	0.68	54.26

图 12　国际医学教育论文 2001—2005 年发文量及被引量的机构分布

7. 国际医学教育论文 2006—2010 年发文量及被引量的机构分布（图 13）

序号	机构	发文量	百分比	序号	机构	被引量	百分比	平均被引量
1	哈佛大学	362	1.42	1	哈佛大学	15 320	1.88	42.32
2	多伦多大学	338	1.33	2	多伦多大学	14 438	1.78	42.72
3	加州大学旧金山分校	272	1.07	3	加州大学旧金山分校	11 032	1.36	40.56
4	华盛顿大学	271	1.07	4	梅奥医学中心	10 368	1.28	47.56
5	梅奥医学中心	218	0.86	5	华盛顿大学	10 367	1.28	38.25
6	密歇根大学	188	0.74	6	西北大学	8818	1.08	70.54
7	约翰斯·霍普金斯大学	186	0.73	7	麦克马斯特大学	7901	0.97	61.25
8	宾夕法尼亚大学	171	0.67	8	宾夕法尼亚大学	6698	0.82	39.17
9	匹兹堡大学	158	0.62	9	约翰斯·霍普金斯大学	6652	0.82	35.76
10	耶鲁大学	152	0.60	10	耶鲁大学	6544	0.80	43.05
11	加州大学洛杉矶分校	143	0.56	11	密歇根大学	6526	0.80	34.71
12	不列颠哥伦比亚大学	135	0.53	12	杜克大学	5843	0.72	43.93
13	杜克大学	133	0.52	13	不列颠哥伦比亚大学	5438	0.67	40.28
14	麦克马斯特大学	129	0.51	14	布莱根妇女医院	5421	0.67	58.29
15	西北大学	125	0.49	15	匹兹堡大学	5261	0.65	33.30

图 13　国际医学教育论文 2006—2010 年发文量及被引量的机构分布

8. 国际医学教育论文 2011—2015 年发文量及被引量的机构分布（图 14）

序号	机构	发文量	百分比	序号	机构	被引量	百分比	平均被引量
1	多伦多大学	531	1.37	1	多伦多大学	14 702	1.60	27.69
2	哈佛大学	520	1.34	2	哈佛大学	14 480	1.58	27.85
3	华盛顿大学	435	1.12	3	梅奥医学中心	13 795	1.51	42.71
4	加州大学旧金山分校	359	0.93	4	加州大学旧金山分校	12 637	1.38	35.20
5	梅奥医学中心	323	0.84	5	华盛顿大学	12 629	1.38	29.03
6	马斯特里赫特大学	271	0.70	6	马斯特里赫特大学	9730	1.06	35.90
7	密歇根大学	270	0.70	7	密歇根大学	8207	0.90	30.40
8	宾夕法尼亚大学	245	0.63	8	西北大学	7675	0.84	33.52
9	不列颠哥伦比亚大学	236	0.61	9	耶鲁大学	7412	0.81	34.80
10	西北大学	229	0.59	10	不列颠哥伦比亚大学	7317	0.80	31.00
11	约翰斯·霍普金斯大学	229	0.59	11	斯坦福大学	6415	0.70	28.51
12	斯坦福大学	225	0.58	12	宾夕法尼亚大学	6231	0.68	25.43
13	耶鲁大学	213	0.55	13	麻省总医院	6016	0.66	28.92
14	杜克大学	208	0.54	14	布莱根妇女医院	5763	0.63	31.49
15	麻省总医院	208	0.54	15	邓迪大学	5605	0.61	59.00

图 14　国际医学教育论文 2011—2015 年发文量及被引量的机构分布

9. 国际医学教育论文 2016—2020 年发文量及被引量的机构分布（图 15）

序号	机构	发文量	百分比	序号	机构	被引量	百分比	平均被引量
1	哈佛大学医学院	642	1.18	1	哈佛大学医学院	7023	1.28	10.94
2	多伦多大学	627	1.15	2	多伦多大学	6911	1.26	11.02
3	华盛顿大学	559	1.03	3	加州大学旧金山分校	6698	1.22	13.24
4	加州大学旧金山分校	506	0.93	4	华盛顿大学	6651	1.21	11.90
5	密歇根大学	463	0.85	5	梅奥医学中心	5420	0.99	13.55
6	梅奥医学中心	400	0.73	6	密歇根大学	5142	0.94	11.11
7	宾夕法尼亚大学	383	0.70	7	宾夕法尼亚大学	5110	0.93	13.34
8	斯坦福大学	371	0.68	8	斯坦福大学	4565	0.83	12.30
9	马斯特里赫特大学	342	0.63	9	西北大学	4374	0.80	13.71
10	西北大学	319	0.59	10	渥太华大学	4209	0.77	14.08
11	约翰斯·霍普金斯大学	305	0.56	11	马斯特里赫特大学	4107	0.75	12.01
12	渥太华大学	299	0.55	12	麦吉尔大学	3610	0.66	14.50
13	科罗拉多大学	287	0.53	13	约翰斯·霍普金斯大学	3496	0.64	11.46
14	不列颠哥伦比亚大学	273	0.50	14	明尼苏达大学	3413	0.62	14.46
15	麻省总医院	263	0.48	15	麻省总医院	3266	0.59	12.42

图 15　国际医学教育论文 2016—2020 年发文量及被引量的机构分布

10. 国际医学教育论文 2001—2020 年发文量及被引量的机构分布排名分析（图 16）

序号	机构	发文量排名 2001—2005	2006—2010	2011—2015	2016—2020	序号	机构	被引量排名 2001—2005	2006—2010	2011—2015	2016—2020
1	哈佛大学医学院	444	655	1101	1	1	哈佛大学医学院	987	1266	293	1
2	多伦多大学	1	2	1	2	2	多伦多大学	3	2	1	2
3	华盛顿大学	4	4	3	3	3	加州大学旧金山分校	6	3	4	3
4	加州大学旧金山分校	5	3	4	4	4	华盛顿大学	2	5	5	4
5	密歇根大学	6	6	6	5	5	梅奥医学中心	41	4	3	5
6	梅奥医学中心	40	5	5	6	6	密歇根大学	9	11	7	6
7	宾夕法尼亚大学	7	8	8	7	7	宾夕法尼亚大学	8	8	12	7
8	斯坦福大学	19	19	12	8	8	斯坦福大学	20	17	11	8
9	马斯特里赫特大学	37	25	6	9	9	西北大学	7	6	9	9
10	西北大学	13	15	10	10	10	渥太华大学	85	28	22	10
11	约翰斯·霍普金斯大学	12	7	10	11	11	马斯特里赫特大学	33	21	6	11
12	渥太华大学	75	49	23	12	12	麦吉尔大学	17	19	19	12
13	科罗拉多大学	17	28	27	13	13	约翰斯·霍普金斯大学	13	9	16	13
14	不列颠哥伦比亚大学	48	12	9	14	14	明尼苏达大学	55	22	29	14
15	麻省总医院	24	23	14	15	15	麻省总医院	23	16	13	15
16	哈佛大学	2	1	2	70	16	哈佛大学	1	1	2	42

图 16　国际医学教育论文 2001—2020 年发文量及被引量的机构分布排名分析

11. 国际医学教育论文 2001—2005 年发文量及被引量的作者分布（图 17）

序号	高发文作者	所在机构	发文量	序号	高被引作者	所在机构	被引量	平均被引量
1	van der Vleuten, Cees P. M.	马斯特里赫特大学	63	1	van der Vleuten, Cees P. M.	马斯特里赫特大学	3952	62.73
2	Regehr, Glenn	多伦多大学	39	2	Regehr, Glenn	多伦多大学	2891	74.13
3	Scherpbier, Albert J. J. A.	马斯特里赫特大学	36	3	McGaghie, William C.	西北大学	2484	177.43
4	Boulet, John R.	外国医学毕业生教育委员会	30	4	A. G. Gallagher	埃默里大学	2432	304.00
5	Mohammadreza Hojat	托马斯·杰斐逊大学	21	5	John W. Cronin	布莱根妇女医院	2402	800.67
6	Geoffrey R. Norman	麦克马斯特大学	21	6	Charles A. Czeisler	布莱根妇女医院	2402	800.67
7	Cees van der Vleuten	马斯特里赫特大学	20	7	R. M. Satava	华盛顿大学	2327	387.83
8	Diana H.J.M. Dolmans	马斯特里赫特大学	19	8	Kevin W. Eva	麦克马斯特大学	2243	160.21
9	Judy A Shea	宾夕法尼亚大学	19	9	S. Barry Issenberg	迈阿密大学	2178	272.25
10	Darzi, Ara	帝国理工学院	18	10	Mohammadreza Hojat	托马斯·杰斐逊大学	2159	102.81
11	Joseph S. Gonnella	托马斯·杰斐逊大学	18	11	David Lee Gordon	迈阿密大学	2114	352.33
12	Scott M. Wright	约翰斯·霍普金斯大学	18	12	Emil R. Petrusa	杜克大学	2055	342.50
13	Tim Dornan	曼彻斯特大学	17	13	Joel T. Katz	布莱根妇女医院	1909	477.25
14	Ronald M. Harden	邓迪大学	17	14	Ross J. Scalese	迈阿密大学	1898	1898.00
15	Clarence D. Kreiter	爱荷华大学	17	15	William T. Branch Jr	埃默里大学	1891	145.46

图 17　国际医学教育论文 2001—2005 年发文量及被引量的作者分布

12. 国际医学教育论文 2006—2010 年发文量及被引量的作者分布（图 18）

序号	高发文作者	所在机构	发文量	序号	高被引作者	所在机构	被引量	平均被引量
1	van der Vleuten, Cees P. M.	马斯特里赫特大学	50	1	McGaghie, William C.	西北大学	4292	171.68
2	Scherpbier, Albert J. J. A.	马斯特里赫特大学	39	2	Wayne, Diane B.	西北大学	2639	138.89
3	Durning, Steven J.	健康科学统一服务大学	32	3	Shanafelt, Tait D.	梅奥医学中心	2467	224.27
4	Cook, David A.	梅奥医学中心	31	4	Frank, Jason R.	渥太华大学	2434	270.44
5	Darzi, Ara	帝国理工学院	31	5	Norman, Geoff	麦克马斯特大学	2414	142.00
6	Boulet, John R.	国际医学教育和研究促进基金会	28	6	Sloan, Jeff A.	梅奥医学中心	2410	301.25
7	Dubrowski, Adam	多伦多大学	28	7	Ten Cate, Olle	乌得勒支大学医学中心	2325	166.07
8	Muijtjens, Arno M. M.	马斯特里赫特大学	28	8	West, Colin P.	梅奥医学中心	2173	127.82
9	Eva, Kevin W.	麦克马斯特大学	26	9	Cook, David A.	梅奥医学中心	2136	68.90
10	Beckman, Thomas J.	梅奥医学中心	25	10	van der Vleuten, Cees P. M.	马斯特里赫特大学	2056	41.12
11	McGaghie, William C.	西北大学	25	11	Darzi, Ara	帝国理工学院	2005	64.68
12	Regehr, Glenn	不列颠哥伦比亚大学	25	12	Barsuk, Jeffrey H.	西北大学	1954	217.11
13	Aggarwal, Rajesh	帝国理工学院	24	13	Regehr, Glenn	不列颠哥伦比亚大学	1853	74.12
14	Cohen-Schotanus, Janke	格罗宁根大学	24	14	Aggarwal, Rajesh	帝国理工学院	1852	77.17
15	Holmboe, Eric S.	美国内科委员会	24	15	Holmboe, Eric S.	美国内科学委员会	1755	73.13

图 18　国际医学教育论文 2006—2010 年发文量及被引量的作者分布

13. 国际医学教育论文 2011—2015 年发文量及被引量的作者分布（图 19）

序号	高发文作者	所在机构	发文量		序号	高被引作者	所在机构	被引量	平均被引量
1	van der Vleuten, Cees P. M.	马斯特里赫特大学	85		1	Cook, David A.	梅奥医学中心	4188	130.88
2	Durning, Steven J.	健康科学统一服务大学	61		2	van der Vleuten, Cees P. M.	马斯特里赫特大学	3715	43.71
3	van der Vleuten, Cees	马斯特里赫特大学	47		3	Reed, Darcy A.	梅奥医学中心	3348	152.18
4	Artino, Anthony R., Jr.	健康科学统一服务大学	46		4	Guthrie, Bruce	邓迪大学	3102	1034.00
5	Scherpbier, Albert J. J. A.	马斯特里赫特大学	46		5	Norbury, Michael	邓迪大学	3095	1547.50
6	Darzi, Ara	帝国理工学院	41		6	Barnett, Karen	邓迪大学	3075	3075.00
7	Aggarwal, Rajesh	麦吉尔大学	40		7	Mercer, Stewart W.	格拉斯哥大学	3075	3075.00
8	Dornan, Tim	马斯特里赫特大学	36		8	Watt, Graham	格拉斯哥大学	3075	3075.00
9	Ringsted, Charlotte	多伦多大学	35		9	Wyke, Sally	格拉斯哥大学	3075	3075.00
10	Regehr, Glenn	不列颠哥伦比亚大学	33		10	O'Brien, Bridget C.	加州大学旧金山分校	2632	219.33
11	Cook, David A.	梅奥医学中心	32		11	Beckman, Thomas J.	梅奥医学中心	2534	133.37
12	Scheele, Fedde	阿姆斯特丹自由大学	30		12	Harris, Ilene B.	伊利诺伊大学	2407	401.17
13	Holmboe, Eric S.	毕业后医学教育认证委员会	29		13	Shanafelt, Tait D.	梅奥医学中心	2361	147.56
14	Lingard, Lorelei	西安大略大学	29		14	McGaghie, William C.	芝加哥洛约拉大学	2149	85.96
15	Ahmed, Kamran	伦敦国王学院	28		15	West, Colin P.	梅奥医学中心	2071	115.06

图 19　国际医学教育论文 2011—2015 年发文量及被引量的作者分布

14. 国际医学教育论文 2016—2020 年发文量及被引量的作者分布（图 20）

序号	高发文作者	所在机构	发文量		序号	高被引作者	所在机构	被引量	平均被引量
1	Durning, Steven J.	健康科学统一服务大学	64		1	Ten Cate, Olle	乌得勒支大学医学中心	1467	22.92
2	Park, Yoon Soo	伊利诺伊大学	64		2	Englander, Robert	明尼苏达大学	1145	44.04
3	Ten Cate, Olle	乌得勒支大学医学中心	64		3	Carraccio, Carol	美国儿科学委员会	967	37.19
4	Santen, Sally A.	弗吉尼亚联邦大学	50		4	Durning, Steven J.	健康科学统一服务大学	925	14.45
5	O'Sullivan, Patricia S.	加州大学旧金山分校	44		5	Frank, Jason R.	渥太华大学	913	36.52
6	Konge, Lars	哥本哈根大学	42		6	Varpio, Lara	健康科学统一服务大学	873	29.10
7	van der Vleuten, Cees	马斯特里赫特大学	42		7	Bilimoria, Karl Y.	西北大学	843	33.72
8	Teunissen, Pim W.	马斯特里赫特大学	40		8	Holmboe, Eric S.	毕业后医学教育认证委员会	805	32.20
9	Cleland, Jennifer	南洋理工大学	39		9	Sherbino, Jonathan	麦克马斯特大学	786	26.20
10	Tekian, Ara	伊利诺伊大学	39		10	van der Vleuten, Cees P. M.	马斯特里赫特大学	735	18.85
11	van der Vleuten, Cees P. M.	马斯特里赫特大学	39		11	O'Sullivan, Patricia S.	加州大学旧金山分校	668	15.18
12	Schwartz, Alan	伊利诺伊大学	37		12	Yang, Anthony D.	西北大学	652	40.75
13	Lingard, Lorelei	西安大略大学	36		13	Konge, Lars	哥本哈根大学	626	14.90
14	Sandhu, Gurjit	密歇根大学	36		14	Touchie, Claire	渥太华大学	625	39.06
15	Regehr, Glenn	不列颠哥伦比亚大学	33		15	Dyrbye, Liselotte N.	梅奥医学中心	623	38.94

图 20　国际医学教育论文 2016—2020 年发文量及被引量的作者分布

15. 国际医学教育论文 2001—2020 年发文量及被引量的作者分布排名分析（图 21）

作者	发文量排名				作者	被引量排名			
	2001—2005	2006—2010	2011—2015	2016—2020		2001—2005	2006—2010	2011—2015	2016—2020
Durning, Steven J.	39	3	2	1	Ten Cate, Olle	1649	7	26	1
Park, Yoon Soo	—	—	35	1	Englander, Robert	161	14 441	342	2
Ten Cate, Olle	799	62	35	1	Carraccio, Carol	139	237	2605	3
Santen, Sally A.	799	2872	103	4	Durning, Steven J.	542	51	17	4
O'Sullivan, Patricia S.	150	18	35	5	Frank, Jason R.	3581	4	671	5
Konge, Lars	—	—	43	6	Varpio, Lara	—	1564	1047	6
van der Vleuten, Cees	7	18	3	6	Bilimoria, Karl Y.	—	4386	2320	7
Teunissen, Pim W.	—	118	31	8	Holmboe, Eric S.	78	14	35	8
Cleland, Jennifer	799	41	120	9	Sherbino, Jonathan	—	49	71	9
Tekian, Ara	799	592	54	9	van der Vleuten, Cees P. M.	1	10	2	10
van der Vleuten, Cees P. M.	1	1	1	9	O'Sullivan, Patricia S.	875	134	80	11
Schwartz, Alan	469	285	144	12	Yang, Anthony D.	—	—	18 374	12
Lingard, Lorelei	16	36	13	13	Konge, Lars	—	—	266	13
Sandhu, Gurjit	—	—	4662	13	Touchie, Claire	4812	10 261	3316	14
Regehr, Glenn	2	10	10	15	Dyrbye, Liselotte N.	—	47	18	15

图 21　国际医学教育论文 2001—2020 年发文量及被引量的作者分布排名分析

（二）研究热点

1. 国际医学教育论文 2001—2005 年高频主题词分布（图 22 ）

序号	主题词	频次	百分比	序号	主题词	频次	百分比
1	Internship and Residency	1853	6.04	21	Physician-Patient Relations	231	0.75
2	Education, Medical, Undergraduate	1315	4.28	22	Computer-Assisted Instruction	208	0.68
3	Clinical Competence	1140	3.71	23	Emergency Medicine	208	0.68
4	Education, Medical	1052	3.43	24	Career Choice	207	0.67
5	Students, Medical	757	2.47	25	Physicians	204	0.66
6	Education, Medical, Graduate	756	2.46	26	Internet	198	0.65
7	Education, Medical, Continuing	648	2.11	27	Psychiatry	194	0.63
8	Teaching	566	1.84	28	Practice Patterns, Physicians'	191	0.62
9	Family Practice	552	1.80	29	Communication	173	0.56
10	Curriculum	540	1.76	30	Physicians, Family	172	0.56
11	Educational Measurement	505	1.65	31	Primary Health Care	155	0.51
12	Attitude of Health Personnel	493	1.61	32	Radiology	150	0.49
13	General Surgery	484	1.58	33	Specialization	150	0.49
14	Pediatrics	313	1.02	34	Professional Competence	138	0.45
15	Faculty, Medical	289	0.94	35	Learning	134	0.44
16	Schools, Medical	281	0.92	36	Academic Medical Centers	128	0.42
17	Problem-Based Learning	277	0.90	37	Obstetrics	127	0.41
18	Internal Medicine	263	0.86	38	Gynecology	126	0.41
19	Clinical Clerkship	250	0.81	39	Health Knowledge, Attitudes, Practice	126	0.41
20	Medical Staff, Hospital	243	0.79	40	Laparoscopy	126	0.41

图 22　国际医学教育论文 2001—2005 年高频主题词分布

2. 国际医学教育论文 2006—2010 年高频主题词分布（图 23 ）

序号	主题词	频次	百分比	序号	主题词	频次	百分比
1	Internship and Residency	2945	5.82	21	Computer-Assisted Instruction	361	0.71
2	Clinical Competence	1932	3.82	22	Career Choice	355	0.70
3	Education, Medical	1566	3.09	23	Emergency Medicine	320	0.63
4	Education, Medical, Undergraduate	1558	3.08	24	Internet	306	0.60
5	Students, Medical	1480	2.92	25	Physician-Patient Relations	297	0.59
6	Education, Medical, Graduate	1462	2.89	26	Learning	295	0.58
7	Education, Medical, Continuing	1053	2.08	27	Medical Staff, Hospital	286	0.56
8	Teaching	904	1.79	28	Health Knowledge, Attitudes, Practice	284	0.56
9	Curriculum	895	1.77	29	Laparoscopy	281	0.56
10	Educational Measurement	768	1.52	30	Communication	266	0.53
11	General Surgery	757	1.50	31	Clinical Clerkship	259	0.51
12	Attitude of Health Personnel	731	1.44	32	Professional Competence	254	0.50
13	Schools, Medical	548	1.08	33	Practice Patterns, Physicians'	231	0.46
14	Faculty, Medical	497	0.98	34	Academic Medical Centers	213	0.42
15	Pediatrics	462	0.91	35	Computer Simulation	211	0.42
16	Family Practice	425	0.84	36	Physicians, Family	210	0.41
17	Physicians	422	0.83	37	Anesthesiology	209	0.41
18	Internal Medicine	409	0.81	38	Anatomy	207	0.41
19	Psychiatry	392	0.77	39	Patient Simulation	202	0.40
20	Problem-Based Learning	362	0.72	40	Biomedical Research	197	0.39

图 23　国际医学教育论文 2006—2010 年高频主题词分布

3. 国际医学教育论文 2011—2015 年高频主题词分布（图 24）

序号	主题词	频次	百分比	序号	主题词	频次	百分比
1	Internship and Residency	3947	5.91	21	Emergency Medicine	403	0.60
2	Clinical Competence	2827	4.24	22	Health Knowledge, Attitudes, Practice	397	0.59
3	Students, Medical	2237	3.35	23	Psychiatry	393	0.59
4	Education, Medical	1960	2.94	24	Computer-Assisted Instruction	389	0.58
5	Education, Medical, Undergraduate	1943	2.91	25	Laparoscopy	387	0.58
6	Education, Medical, Graduate	1845	2.76	26	Internal Medicine	367	0.55
7	Education, Medical, Continuing	1205	1.81	27	Clinical Clerkship	362	0.54
8	Curriculum	1161	1.74	28	Problem-Based Learning	356	0.53
9	Educational Measurement	1070	1.60	29	Physician-Patient Relations	332	0.50
10	Attitude of Health Personnel	976	1.46	30	Anatomy	319	0.48
11	Teaching	883	1.32	31	Communication	319	0.48
12	General Surgery	877	1.31	32	Internet	315	0.47
13	Physicians	696	1.04	33	Radiology	308	0.46
14	Faculty, Medical	606	0.91	34	Practice Patterns, Physicians'	293	0.44
15	Pediatrics	560	0.84	35	Medical Staff, Hospital	279	0.42
16	Schools, Medical	554	0.83	36	Biomedical Research	277	0.42
17	Career Choice	474	0.71	37	Professional Competence	271	0.41
18	Learning	452	0.68	38	Anesthesiology	252	0.38
19	Computer Simulation	430	0.64	39	Fellowships and Scholarships	245	0.37
20	Family Practice	417	0.62	40	Quality Improvement	237	0.36

图 24 国际医学教育论文 2011—2015 年高频主题词分布

4. 国际医学教育论文 2016—2020 年高频主题词分布（图 25）

序号	主题词	频次	百分比	序号	主题词	频次	百分比
1	Internship and Residency	5532	7.04	21	Emergency Medicine	447	0.57
2	Clinical Competence	3232	4.11	22	Clinical Clerkship	433	0.55
3	Students, Medical	3193	4.06	23	Fellowships and Scholarships	432	0.55
4	Education, Medical, Graduate	2360	3.00	24	Psychiatry	421	0.54
5	Education, Medical, Undergraduate	2342	2.98	25	Anatomy	420	0.53
6	Education, Medical	2145	2.73	26	Problem-Based Learning	419	0.53
7	Curriculum	1578	2.01	27	Internal Medicine	413	0.53
8	Educational Measurement	1147	1.46	28	Health Knowledge, Attitudes, Practice	394	0.50
9	General Surgery	1059	1.35	29	Family Practice	368	0.47
10	Physicians	979	1.25	30	Communication	362	0.46
11	Simulation Training	961	1.22	31	Orthopedics	343	0.44
12	Attitude of Health Personnel	892	1.13	32	Laparoscopy	341	0.43
13	Education, Medical, Continuing	847	1.08	33	Radiology	336	0.43
14	Faculty, Medical	638	0.81	34	Burnout, Professional	332	0.42
15	Pediatrics	593	0.75	35	Quality Improvement	331	0.42
16	Learning	580	0.74	36	Health Personnel	328	0.42
17	Teaching	578	0.74	37	Biomedical Research	326	0.41
18	Schools, Medical	561	0.71	38	Computer-Assisted Instruction	313	0.40
19	Career Choice	558	0.71	39	Competency-Based Education	311	0.40
20	Surgeons	453	0.58	40	Otolaryngology	298	0.38

图 25 国际医学教育论文 2016—2020 年高频主题词分布

5. 国际医学教育论文 2001—2020 年高频主题词分布排名分析（图 26）

主题词	频次排名				主题词	频次排名			
	2001—2005	2006—2010	2011—2015	2016—2020		2001—2005	2006—2010	2011—2015	2016—2020
Internship and Residency	1	1	1	1	Emergency Medicine	23	23	21	21
Clinical Competence	3	2	2	2	Clinical Clerkship	19	31	27	22
Students, Medical	5	2	3	3	Fellowships and Scholarships	56	43	39	23
Education, Medical, Graduate	6	3	6	4	Psychiatry	27	19	23	24
Education, Medical, Undergraduate	2	4	5	5	Anatomy	50	38	30	25
Education, Medical	4	3	4	6	Problem-Based Learning	17	20	28	26
Curriculum	10	9	8	7	Internal Medicine	18	18	26	27
Educational Measurement	11	10	9	8	Health Knowledge, Attitudes, Practice	39	28	22	28
General Surgery	13	11	12	9	Family Practice	9	16	20	29
Physicians	25	17	13	10	Communication	29	30	31	30
Simulation Training	—	—	87	11	Orthopedics	68	46	48	31
Attitude of Health Personnel	12	12	10	12	Laparoscopy	40	29	25	32
Education, Medical, Continuing	7	7	7	13	Radiology	32	44	33	33
Faculty, Medical	15	14	14	14	Burnout, Professional	185	148	118	34
Pediatrics	14	15	15	15	Quality Improvement	—	561	40	35
Learning	35	26	18	16	Health Personnel	102	71	43	36
Teaching	8	8	11	17	Biomedical Research	58	40	36	37
Schools, Medical	16	13	16	18	Computer-Assisted Instruction	22	21	24	38
Career Choice	24	22	17	19	Competency-Based Education	59	41	51	39
Surgeons	—	—	166	20	Otolaryngology	112	83	49	40

图 26　国际医学教育论文 2001—2020 年高频主题词分布排名分析

6. 国际医学教育论文 2001—2005 年高频主题词聚类（图 27）

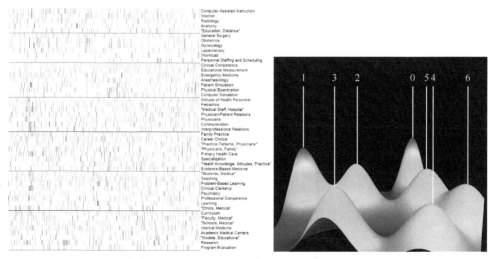

图 27　国际医学教育论文 2001—2005 年高频主题词聚类

注：右图中数字表示高频主题词聚类所形成的主题类别。

通过高频主题词聚类分析，2001—2005 年国际医学教育研究主题涵盖以下 6 个主要方面：

（1）基于互联网的医学课程教学模式和方法改革研究。

（2）住院医师工作负荷及其与工作满意度、医疗服务质量的关系研究。

（3）医学模拟教学在临床技能考核与评价中的应用。

（4）循证医学及其在临床实践中的应用。

（5）临床教师、住院医师和医学生的职业精神研究。

（6）其他类，包括对住院医师项目和跨学科课程的评价研究。

7. 国际医学教育论文 2006—2010 年高频主题词聚类（图 28）

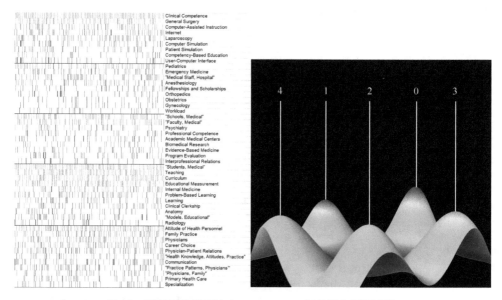

图 28　国际医学教育论文 2006—2010 年高频主题词聚类

注：右图中数字表示高频主题词聚类所形成的主题类别。

通过高频主题词聚类分析，2006—2010 年国际医学教育研究主题涵盖以下 5 个主要方面：

（1）医学模拟教学在临床技能培训中的应用及效果评价研究。

（2）住院医师规范化培训制度改革研究，特别是工作负荷合理化与薪酬待遇提升研究。

（3）临床医师和医学生非技术性能力培养与提升研究。

（4）课程教学与评价的理论、模式和方法改革研究。

（5）其他类，包括医师和医学生的专业选择、初级卫生保健质量提升研究。

8. 国际医学教育论文 2011—2015 年高频主题词聚类（图 29）

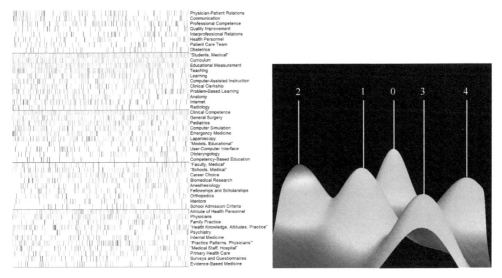

图 29　国际医学教育论文 2011—2015 年高频主题词聚类

注：右图中数字表示高频主题词聚类所形成的主题类别。

通过高频主题词聚类分析，2011—2015 年国际医学教育研究主题涵盖以下 5 个主要方面：

（1）临床人际沟通技能与团队合作能力培养研究。

（2）基于互联网的医学课程教学与评价研究。

（3）医学模拟教学在临床技能培训中的应用。

（4）临床教师和医学生学术职业发展以及影响因素研究。

（5）循证医学及其在临床实践中的应用。

9. 国际医学教育论文 2016—2020 年高频主题词聚类（图 30）

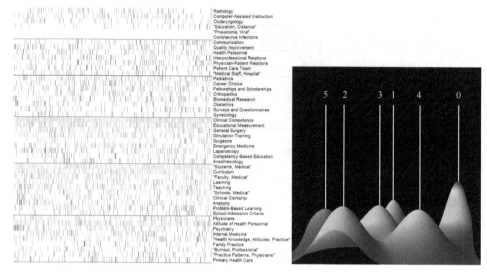

图 30　国际医学教育论文 2016—2020 年高频主题词聚类

注：右图中数字表示高频主题词聚类所形成的主题类别。

通过高频主题词聚类分析，2016—2020 年国际医学教育研究主题涵盖以下 6 个主要方面：

（1）在新冠肺炎疫情影响下，医学教学模式和方法改革研究。

（2）跨专业医疗团队中的沟通研究。

（3）基于医学模拟教学的临床技能培训与评价研究。

（4）以学生为中心的教学研究。

（5）医师职业倦怠、影响因素及干预研究。

（6）其他类，包括职业选择、绩效分配等。

三、全球医学教育教学研究专题分析

（一）研究方法

1. 检索策略

MeSH 主题词 "Education, Medical" ＋ JCR 数据库中教育门类下 10 种医学教育期刊（*Academic Medicine / Medical Education / Medical Teacher / BMC Medical Education / Journal of Surgical Education / Advances in Health Sciences Education / Teaching and Learning in Medicine / Medical Education Online / Anatomical Sciences Education / Academic Psychiatry*）AND MeSH 主题词 "Teaching"。

2. 统计年限

2012 年 1 月 1 日至 2021 年 12 月 31 日。

3. 分析方法

文献概览采用可视化分析工具 CiteSpace 对高发文量国家、机构、作者进行统计；对近 10 年纳入文献（2012—2021）的主要主题词进行高频主题词聚类分析；对 2011—2020 年纳入文献的高被引文献进行共被引聚类分析。

（二）文献概览及研究前沿

1. 全球医学教育教学研究 2012—2021 年发文量国家 / 地区分布（图 31）

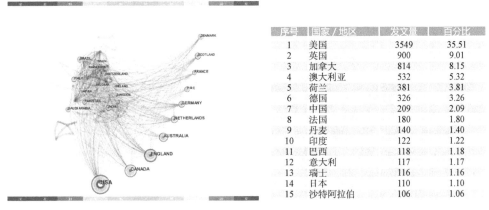

序号	国家 / 地区	发文量	百分比
1	美国	3549	35.51
2	英国	900	9.01
3	加拿大	814	8.15
4	澳大利亚	532	5.32
5	荷兰	381	3.81
6	德国	326	3.26
7	中国	209	2.09
8	法国	180	1.80
9	丹麦	140	1.40
10	印度	122	1.22
11	巴西	118	1.18
12	意大利	117	1.17
13	瑞士	116	1.16
14	日本	110	1.10
15	沙特阿拉伯	106	1.06

图 31　全球医学教育教学研究 2012—2021 年发文量国家 / 地区分布

注：左图中的 CiteSpace 发文年环代表着文献的发文历史，年轮的整体大小反映某个国家 / 地区的累计发文量。发文年环的颜色代表相应的发文时间。一个年轮厚度和相应的时间分区内发文数量成正比。不同国家 / 地区间的连线表示对应的论文合著关系。引文年环类同。

2. 全球医学教育教学研究 2012—2021 年发文量机构分布（图 32）

序号	机构	发文量	百分比
1	多伦多大学	255	1.32
2	马斯特里赫特大学	177	0.91
3	梅奥医学中心	148	0.76
4	加州大学旧金山分校	145	0.75
5	哈佛大学医学院	131	0.68
6	斯坦福大学	129	0.67
7	哈佛大学	124	0.64
8	密歇根大学	121	0.63
9	西北大学	118	0.61
10	麦吉尔大学	116	0.60
11	华盛顿大学	110	0.57
12	渥太华大学	105	0.54
13	麻省总医院	104	0.54
14	卡尔加里大学	103	0.53
15	纽约大学	99	0.51

图 32　全球医学教育教学研究 2012—2021 年发文量机构分布

注：左图中的 CiteSpace 可视化高发文量机构分布呈现出不同机构的发文量、发文时间和不同机构间紧密的合作状态。

3. 全球医学教育教学研究 2012—2021 年发文量作者分布（图 33）

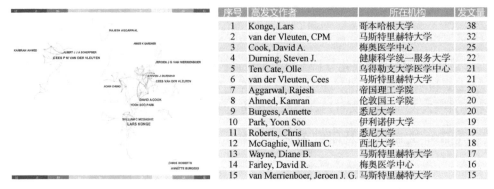

序号	高发文作者	所在机构	发文量
1	Konge, Lars	哥本哈根大学	38
2	van der Vleuten, CPM	马斯特里赫特大学	32
3	Cook, David A.	梅奥医学中心	25
4	Durning, Steven J.	健康科学统一服务大学	22
5	Ten Cate, Olle	乌得勒支大学医学中心	21
6	van der Vleuten, Cees	马斯特里赫特大学	21
7	Aggarwal, Rajesh	帝国理工学院	20
8	Ahmed, Kamran	伦敦国王学院	20
9	Burgess, Annette	悉尼大学	20
10	Park, Yoon Soo	伊利诺伊大学	19
11	Roberts, Chris	悉尼大学	19
12	McGaghie, William C.	西北大学	18
13	Wayne, Diane B.	马斯特里赫特大学	17
14	Farley, David R.	梅奥医学中心	16
15	van Merrienboer, Jeroen J. G.	马斯特里赫特大学	15

图 33　全球医学教育教学研究 2012—2021 年发文量作者分布

注：左图的 CiteSpace 可视化高发文量作者分布呈现出不同作者的发文量、发文时间和不同作者间的相互合作关系。

4. 全球医学教育教学研究 2012—2021 年高频主题词分布（图 34）

序号	主题词	频次	百分比	序号	主题词	频次	百分比
1	Teaching	2308	5.35	21	Pediatrics	297	0.69
2	Education, Medical, Undergraduate	2196	5.09	22	Communication	271	0.63
3	Education, Medical	1958	4.54	23	Education, Distance	263	0.61
4	Internship and Residency	1929	4.47	24	Attitude of Health Personnel	234	0.54
5	Students, Medical	1884	4.37	25	Internet	233	0.54
6	Clinical Competence	1804	4.18	26	Laparoscopy	232	0.54
7	Simulation Training	1563	3.62	27	Schools, Medical	223	0.52
8	Education, Medical, Graduate	1220	2.83	28	Emergency Medicine	220	0.51
9	Problem-Based Learning	1120	2.60	29	Clinical Clerkship	217	0.50
10	Computer-Assisted Instruction	977	2.26	30	Peer Group	196	0.45
11	Curriculum	963	2.23	31	Radiology	185	0.43
12	Learning	601	1.39	32	Anesthesiology	184	0.43
13	Educational Measurement	555	1.29	33	COVID-19	183	0.42
14	Models, Educational	533	1.24	34	Physicians	182	0.42
15	Patient Simulation	490	1.14	35	Internal Medicine	181	0.42
16	Faculty, Medical	475	1.10	36	Physician-Patient Relations	179	0.41
17	General Surgery	459	1.06	37	Interprofessional Relations	156	0.36
18	Education, Medical, Continuing	435	1.01	38	Competency-Based Education	152	0.35
19	Anatomy	407	0.94	39	Patient Care Team	145	0.34
20	Computer Simulation	302	0.70	40	Psychiatry	143	0.33

图 34　全球医学教育教学研究 2012—2021 年高频主题词分布

5. 全球医学教育教学研究 2012—2021 年前 1% 高频被引论文分布（图 35）

序号	高频被引论文	被引频次
1	McLaughlin J E, Roth M T, Glatt D M, et al. The flipped classroom: a course redesign to foster learning and engagement in a health professions school. Acad Med, 2014, 89(2):236-243.	541
2	Motola I, Devine L A, Chung H S, et al. Simulation in healthcare education: a best evidence practical guide. AMEE Guide No. 82. Med Teach, 2013, 35(10):e1511-1530.	381
3	Taylor D C, Hamdy H. Adult learning theories: implications for learning and teaching in medical education: AMEE Guide No. 83. Med Teach, 2013, 35(11):e1561-1572.	347
4	Cook D A, Hamstra S J, Brydges R, et al. Comparative effectiveness of instructional design features in simulation-based education: systematic review and meta-analysis. Med Teach, 2013, 35(1):e867-898.	307
5	Eppich W, Cheng A. Promoting Excellence and Reflective Learning in Simulation (PEARLS): development and rationale for a blended approach to health care simulation debriefing. Simul Healthc, 2015, 10(2):106-115.	286
6	Young J Q, Van Merrienboer J, Durning S, et al. Cognitive Load Theory: implications for medical education: AMEE Guide No. 86. Med Teach, 2014, 36(5):371-384.	282
7	Norman G, Dore K, Grierson L. The minimal relationship between simulation fidelity and transfer of learning. Med Educ, 2012, 46(7):636-647.	281
8	McGaghie W C, Issenberg S B, Barsuk J H, et al. A critical review of simulation-based mastery learning with translational outcomes. Med Educ, 2014, 48(4):375-385.	275
9	Chen F, Lui A M, Martinelli S M. A systematic review of the effectiveness of flipped classrooms in medical education. Med Educ, 2017, 51(6):585-597.	245
10	Hew K F, Lo C K. Flipped classroom improves student learning in health professions education: a meta-analysis. BMC Med Educ, 2018, 18(1):38.	244
11	Ericsson K A. Acquisition and maintenance of medical expertise: a perspective from the expert-performance approach with deliberate practice. Acad Med, 2015, 90(11):1471-1486.	232
12	Moro C, Štromberga Z, Raikos A, et al. The effectiveness of virtual and augmented reality in health sciences and medical anatomy. Anat Sci Educ, 2017, 10(6):549-559.	222
13	Preece D, Williams S B, Lam R, et al. "Let's get physical": advantages of a physical model over 3D computer models and textbooks in learning imaging anatomy. Anat Sci Educ, 2013, 6(4):216-224.	209
14	va K W, Armson H, Holmboe E, et al. Factors influencing responsiveness to feedback: on the interplay between fear, confidence, and reasoning processes. Adv Health Sci Educ Theory Pract, 2012, 17(1):15-26.	209
15	Dedeilia A, Sotiropoulos M G, Hanrahan J G, et al. Medical and surgical education challenges and innovations in the COVID-19 era: a systematic review. In Vivo, 2020, 34(3 Suppl):1603-1611.	173
16	Osseo-Asare A, Balasuriya L, Huot S J, et al. Minority resident physicians' views on the role of race/ethnicity in their training experiences in the workplace. JAMA Network Open, 2018, 1(5):e182723.	160
17	Yammine K, Violato C. A meta-analysis of the educational effectiveness of three-dimensional visualization technologies in teaching anatomy. Anat Sci Educ, 2015, 8(6):525-538.	128
18	Pather N, Blyth P, Chapman J A, et al. Forced disruption of anatomy education in Australia and New Zealand: an acute response to the COVID-19 pandemic. Anat Sci Educ, 2020, 13(3):284-300.	125
19	Pei L, Wu H. Does online learning work better than offline learning in undergraduate medical education? A systematic review and meta-analysis. Med Educ Online, 2019, 24(1):1666538.	122
20	Trelease R B. From chalkboard, slides, and paper to e-learning: How computing technologies have transformed anatomical sciences education. Anat Sci Educ, 2016, 9(6):583-602.	109
21	Al-Balas M, Al-Balas H I, Jaber H M, et al. Distance learning in clinical medical education amid COVID-19 pandemic in Jordan: current situation, challenges, and perspectives. BMC Med Educ, 2020, 20(1):341.	104
22	Kogan M, Klein S E, Hannon C P, et al. Orthopaedic education during the COVID-19 pandemic. J Am Acad Orthop Surg, 2020, 28(11):456-464.	101
23	Gorbanev I, Agudelo-Londoño S, González R A, et al. A systematic review of serious games in medical education: quality of evidence and pedagogical strategy. Med Educ Online, 2018, 23(1):1438718.	74
24	Zhao J, Xu X, Jiang H, et al. The effectiveness of virtual reality-based technology on anatomy teaching: a meta-analysis of randomized controlled studies. BMC Med Educ, 2020, 20(1):127.	38
25	Harmon D J, Attardi S M, Barremkala M, et a;. An analysis of anatomy education before and during COVID-19: May-August 2020. Anat Sci Educ, 2021, 14(2):132-147.	27
26	Jiang Z, Wu H, Cheng H, et al. Twelve tips for teaching medical students online under COVID-19. Med Educ Online, 2021, 26(1):1854066.	22
27	Jack M M, Gattozzi D A, Camarata P J, et al. Live-streaming surgery for medical student education - educational solutions in neurosurgery during the COVID-19 pandemic. J Surg Educ, 2021, 78(1):99-103.	16

图 35　全球医学教育教学研究 2012—2021 年前 1% 高频被引论文分布

6. 全球医学教育教学研究 2012—2021 年高频主题词聚类（图 36）

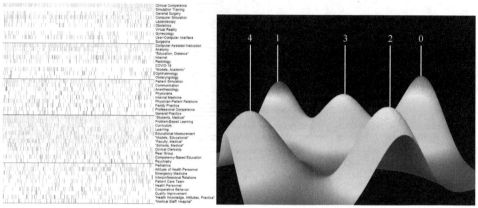

图 36　全球医学教育教学研究 2012—2021 年高频主题词聚类

注：右图中数字表示高频主题词聚类所形成的主题类别。

通过高频主题词聚类分析，全球医学教育教学研究主题涵盖以下 5 个主要方面：

（1）医学模拟教学在临床技能培训中的应用。

（2）在新冠肺炎疫情影响下，医学教学模式与评价方法改革研究。

（3）医患沟通技能培养策略与方法研究。

（4）以胜任力为导向的教学与评价研究。

（5）跨专业教育与团队合作能力培养研究。

7. 全球医学教育教学研究 2011—2020 年引文共被引聚类（图 37）

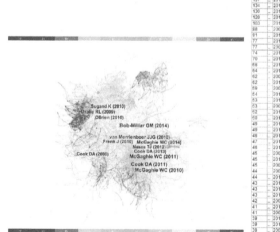

图 37　全球医学教育教学研究 2011—2020 年引文共被引聚类

通过引文共被引聚类分析，近 10 年全球医学教育教学研究高频引文被聚类为以下 7 个主要方面：

（1）医学模拟教学，特别是虚拟病人的研究与实践。

推荐阅读：

[1] McGaghie W C, Issenberg S B, Barsuk J H, et al. A critical review of simulation-based mastery learning with translational outcomes. Med Educ, 2014, 48(4): 375-385.

[2] Cook D A, Hamstra S J, Brydges R, et al. Comparative effectiveness of instructional design features in simulation-based education: systematic review and meta-analysis. Med Teach, 2013, 35(1): e867-898.

[3] Cook D A, Hatala R, Brydges R, et al. Technology-enhanced simulation for health professions education: a systematic review and meta-analysis. JAMA, 2011, 306(9): 978-988.

[4] McGaghie W C, Issenberg S B, Cohen E R, et al. Does simulation-based medical education with deliberate practice yield better results than traditional clinical education? A meta-analytic comparative review of the evidence. Acad Med, 2011, 86(6): 706-711.

[5] McGaghie W C, Issenberg S B, Petrusa E R, et al. A critical review of simulation-based medical education research: 2003-2009. Med Educ, 2010, 44(1): 50-63.

[6] Okuda Y, Bryson E O, DeMaria S Jr, et al. The utility of simulation in medical education: what is the evidence?. Mt Sinai J Med. 2009, 76(4): 330-343.

[7] Cook D A, Erwin P J, Triola M M. Computerized virtual patients in health professions education: a systematic review and meta-analysis. Acad Med, 2010, 85(10): 1589-1602.

[8] Cook D A, Triola M M. Virtual patients: a critical literature review and proposed next steps. Med Educ, 2009, 43(4): 303-311.

（2）强调自我导向学习的教学方法研究。

推荐阅读：

[1] Freeman S, Eddy S L, McDonough M, et al. Active learning increases student performance in science, engineering, and mathematics. Proc Natl Acad Sci U S A, 2014, 111(23): 8410-8415.

[2] McLaughlin J E, Roth M T, Glatt D M, et al. The flipped classroom: a course redesign to foster learning and engagement in a health professions school. Acad Med, 2014, 89(2): 236-243.

[3] Mann K, Gordon J, MacLeod A. Reflection and reflective practice in health professions education: a systematic review. Adv Health Sci Educ Theory Pract, 2009, 14(4): 595-621.

（3）医学教育相关理论的研究、实践与启示。

推荐阅读：

[1] Young J Q, Van Merrienboer J, Durning S, et al. Cognitive Load Theory: implications for medical education: AMEE Guide No. 86. Med Teach, 2014, 36(5): 371-384.

[2] van Merriënboer J J, Sweller J. Cognitive load theory in health professional education: design principles and strategies. Med Educ, 2010, 44(1): 85-93.

[3] Mayer R E. Applying the science of learning to medical education. Med Educ, 2010, 44(6): 543-9.

（4）基于互联网的学习在医学教育中的应用实践。

推荐阅读：

[1] Cook D A, Levinson A J, Garside S, et al. Internet-based learning in the health professions: a meta-analysis. JAMA, 2008, 300(10): 1181-1196.

[2] Cook D A, Levinson A J, Garside S, et al. Instructional design variations in Internet-based learning for health professions education: a systematic review and meta-analysis. Acad Med, 2010, 85(5): 909-922.

[3] Ruiz J G, Mintzer M J, Leipzig R M. The impact of E-learning in medical education. Acad Med, 2006, 81(3): 207-212.

（5）医学教育教学与评价改革研究。

推荐阅读：

[1] Prober C G, Khan S. Medical education reimagined: a call to action. Acad Med, 2013, 88(10): 1407-1410.

[2] Nasca T J, Philibert I, Brigham T, et al. The next GME accreditation system—rationale and benefits. N Engl J Med, 2012, 366(11): 1051-1056.

[3] Irby D M, Cooke M, O'Brien B C. Calls for reform of medical education by the Carnegie Foundation for the Advancement of Teaching: 1910 and 2010. Acad Med, 2010, 85(2): 220-227.

[4] Frenk J, Chen L, Bhutta Z A, et al. Health professionals for a new century: transforming

education to strengthen health systems in an interdependent world. Lancet, 2010, 376(9756): 1923-1958.

（6）外科学技能培训及其与医疗质量的关系研究。

推荐阅读：

[1] Julià D, Gómez N, Codina-Cazador A. Surgical skill and complication rates after bariatric surgery. N Engl J Med, 2014, 370(3): 285.

[2] Mattar S G, Alseidi A A, Jones D B, et al. General surgery residency inadequately prepares trainees for fellowship: results of a survey of fellowship program directors. Ann Surg, 2013, 258(3): 440-449.

[3] Sroka G, Feldman L S, Vassiliou M C, et al. Fundamentals of laparoscopic surgery simulator training to proficiency improves laparoscopic performance in the operating room—a randomized controlled trial. Am J Surg, 2010, 199(1): 115-120.

[4] Reznick R K, MacRae H. Teaching surgical skills—changes in the wind. N Engl J Med, 2006, 355(25): 2664-2669.

（7）解剖学课程的现代化建设，特别是教学模式与方法改革研究。

推荐阅读：

[1] Johnson E O, Charchanti A V, Troupis T G. Modernization of an anatomy class: From conceptualization to implementation. A case for integrated multimodal-multidisciplinary teaching. Anat Sci Educ, 2012, 5(6): 354-366.

[2] Sugand K, Abrahams P, Khurana A. The anatomy of anatomy: a review for its modernization. Anat Sci Educ, 2010, 3(2): 83-93.

[3] Drake R L, McBride J M, Lachman N, et al. Medical education in the anatomical sciences: the winds of change continue to blow. Anat Sci Educ, 2009, 2(6): 253-259.

四、医学教育学科 ESI 排名

ESI（Essential Science Indicators）基本科学指标数据库，是由国际学术信息数据库公司汤森路透推出的衡量科学研究绩效、跟踪科学发展趋势的基本分析评价工具，是基于 Web of Science 引文索引数据库 Science Citation Index（简称 SCI）和 Social Science Citation Index（简称 SSCI）所收录的全球 8500 多种学术期刊的 1000 多万条文献记录而建立的计量分析数据库。ESI 从引文分析的角度，将全部科学分为 22 个专业领域，分别对国家（地区）、研究机构、期刊、论文以及科学家进行统计分析和排序。ESI 是当今世界范围内普遍用以评价高校、学术机构、国家（地区）国际学术水平及影响力的重要评价指标工具之一。

机构发表论文的总被引量是反映一个机构学术能力和影响力的重要指标之一。建设世界一流大学和一流学科是中国做出的重大战略决策，有利于提升一个国家高等教育综合实力和国际竞争力。ESI 前百分之一和千分之一的学科及其相应机构是一流学科和一流大学的重要评价指标之一。因此，我们通过与科睿唯安公司合作，将 ESI 排名的概念引入到了医学教育研究领域，为医学教育学科单独建立 ESI 研究机构统计分析和排序。通过介绍医学教育学科 ESI 机构排名的情况，能够发扬优势也寻找差距，可以为未来的研究和实践工作指明方向。

在《2019 国际医学教育研究前沿报告》中我们首次发布了医学教育的 ESI 机构统计排名，受到了广泛好评和欢迎。在 2022 年我们延续这一内容，更新医学教育研究领域 ESI 机构统计排名，并与前两年发布的 ESI 排名进行了对比，为全球学者提供更好的参考数据。

（一）研究方法

1. 检索策略

MeSH 主题词"Education, Medical"＋JCR 数据库中教育门类下 10 种医学教育期刊（*Academic Medicine / Medical Education / Medical Teacher / BMC Medical Education / Journal of Surgical Education / Advances in Health Sciences Education / Teaching and Learning in Medicine / Medical Education Online / Anatomical Sciences Education / Academic Psychiatry*）。

2. 统计年限

2012 年 1 月 1 日至 2021 年 12 月 31 日。

3. 统计方法

对纳入检索范围论文的总被引用频次进行统计，通过总被引频次反映学术影响力。

（二）医学教育学科 ESI 机构分布

1. ESI 前 1‰机构分布（23/23286）〔图 38〕

序号	ESI 前 1‰机构	所属国家	被引量	发文量	篇均被引量	2020 年 ESI 排名	2021 年 ESI 排名	2022 年 ESI 排名
1	多伦多大学	加拿大	12 845	1535	8.37	1	1	1
2	梅奥医学中心	美国	9776	1025	9.54	3	2	2
3	哈佛大学	美国	9260	799	11.59	2	3	3
4	加州大学旧金山分校	美国	8885	1259	7.06	4	4	4
5	密歇根大学	美国	6993	1112	6.29	7	6	5
6	宾夕法尼亚大学	美国	6691	961	6.96	9	9	6
7	马斯特里赫特大学	荷兰	6408	736	8.71	5	5	7
8	华盛顿大学	美国	6354	879	7.23	13	11	8
9	不列颠哥伦比亚大学	加拿大	6253	686	9.12	8	7	9
10	斯坦福大学	美国	6079	895	6.79	12	12	10
11	渥太华大学	加拿大	6027	625	9.64	10	10	11
12	西北大学	美国	5782	748	7.73	6	8	12
13	约翰斯·霍普金斯大学	美国	5217	769	6.78	14	13	13
14	麻省总医院	美国	5041	707	7.13	17	16	14
15	麦吉尔大学	加拿大	4810	556	8.65	15	15	15
16	麦克马斯特大学	加拿大	4562	574	7.95	11	17	16
17	耶鲁大学	美国	4561	550	8.29	16	14	17
18	范德堡大学	美国	4464	644	6.93	19	20	18
19	杜克大学	美国	4409	619	7.12	18	18	19
20	布莱根妇女医院	美国	4241	603	7.03	20	19	20
21	俄勒冈健康与科学大学	美国	4002	561	7.13	23	22	21
22	卡尔加里大学	加拿大	3898	517	7.54	22	21	22
23	匹兹堡大学	美国	3711	560	6.63	21	23	23

图 38　ESI 前 1‰机构分布

2. 北美洲 ESI 排名前 10 机构分布（图 39）

序号	是否进入ESI 前1%	机构	所属国家	被引量	发文量	篇均被引量	2020 年ESI 排名	2021 年ESI 排名	2022 年ESI 排名
1	√	多伦多大学	加拿大	12 845	1535	8.37	1	1	1
2	√	梅奥医学中心	美国	9776	1025	9.54	3	2	2
3	√	哈佛大学	美国	9260	799	11.59	2	3	3
4	√	加州大学旧金山分校	美国	8885	1259	7.06	4	4	4
5	√	密歇根大学	美国	6993	1112	6.29	7	6	5
6	√	宾夕法尼亚大学	美国	6691	961	6.96	9	9	6
7	√	华盛顿大学	美国	6354	879	7.23	13	11	8
8	√	不列颠哥伦比亚大学	加拿大	6253	686	9.12	8	7	9
9	√	斯坦福大学	美国	6079	895	6.79	12	12	10
10	√	渥太华大学	加拿大	6027	625	9.64	10	10	11

图 39 北美洲 ESI 排名前 10 机构分布

3. 欧洲 ESI 排名前 10 机构分布（图 40）

序号	是否进入ESI 前1%	机构	所属国家	被引量	发文量	篇均被引量	2020 年ESI 排名	2021 年ESI 排名	2022 年ESI 排名
1	√	马斯特里赫特大学	荷兰	6408	736	8.71	5	5	7
2	√	邓迪大学	英国	3294	197	16.72	29	31	29
3	√	帝国理工学院	英国	2386	215	11.10	28	40	48
4	√	格拉斯哥大学	英国	2363	105	22.50	58	54	49
5	√	乌得勒支大学医学中心	荷兰	2101	213	9.86	54	55	53
6	√	伦敦大学学院	英国	1938	328	5.91	64	65	61
7	√	伦敦国王学院	英国	1862	342	5.44	67	64	67
8	√	阿姆斯特丹大学	荷兰	1853	200	9.27	57	61	70
9	√	拉德堡德大学	荷兰	1459	208	7.01	88	84	84
10	√	牛津大学	英国	1334	275	4.85	97	87	91

图 40 欧洲 ESI 排名前 10 机构分布

4. 大洋洲 ESI 排名前 10 机构分布（图 41）

序号	是否进入ESI前1%	机构	所属国家	被引量	发文量	篇均被引量	2020年ESI排名	2021年ESI排名	2022年ESI排名
1	√	墨尔本大学	澳大利亚	2807	337	8.33	42	39	39
2	√	悉尼大学	澳大利亚	2754	373	7.38	44	41	40
3	√	蒙纳士大学	澳大利亚	2658	401	6.63	48	43	44
4	√	弗林德斯大学	澳大利亚	1709	199	8.59	79	73	75
5	√	昆士兰大学	澳大利亚	1626	242	6.72	69	75	78
6	√	奥塔哥大学	新西兰	911	165	5.52	190	153	139
7	√	西澳大利亚大学	澳大利亚	883	142	6.22	177	139	144
8	√	奥克兰大学	新西兰	856	161	5.32	141	129	147
9	√	阿德莱德大学	澳大利亚	771	127	6.07	203	163	159
10	√	格里菲斯大学	澳大利亚	717	110	6.52	247	195	171

图 41　大洋洲 ESI 排名前 10 机构分布

5. 亚洲 ESI 排名前 10 机构分布（图 42）

序号	是否进入ESI前1%	机构	所属国家	被引量	发文量	篇均被引量	2020年ESI排名	2021年ESI排名	2022年ESI排名
1	√	沙特国王大学	沙特阿拉伯	977	151	6.47	165	132	124
2	√	新加坡国立大学	新加坡	778	174	4.47	265	162	157
3	√	香港大学	中国	566	91	6.22	239	220	209
4		延世大学	韩国	419	44	9.52	298	258	269
5		阿卜杜勒·阿齐兹国王大学	沙特阿拉伯	330	85	3.88	449	381	326
6		沙特国王健康科学大学	沙特阿拉伯	326	57	5.72	389	339	327
7		新加坡国立大学医院	新加坡	321	72	4.46	427	334	332
8		全印医学科学学院	印度	315	108	2.92	652	433	344
9		香港中文大学	中国	297	45	6.60	321	428	368
10		台湾大学	中国	284	60	4.73	395	375	383

图 42　亚洲 ESI 排名前 10 机构分布

6. 非洲 ESI 排名前 10 机构分布（图 43）

序号	是否进入ESI 前1%	机构	所属国家	被引量	发文量	篇均被引量	2020 年ESI 排名	2021 年ESI 排名	2022 年ESI 排名
1	√	开普敦大学	南非	578	103	5.61	153	125	206
2		斯坦陵布什大学	南非	499	51	9.78	227	218	238
3		马凯雷雷大学	乌干达	349	56	6.23	212	211	313
4		夸祖鲁·纳塔尔大学	南非	298	69	4.32	413	393	366
5		加纳大学	加纳	276	19	14.53	467	416	394
6		马拉维大学	马拉维	217	33	6.58	378	329	494
7		西开普大学	南非	194	21	9.24	723	598	538
8		威特沃特斯兰德大学	南非	157	54	2.91	761	696	660
9		穆希比利医科大学	坦桑尼亚	149	26	5.73	933	800	684
10		内罗毕大学	肯尼亚	149	27	5.52	963	811	684

图 43　非洲 ESI 排名前 10 机构分布

7. 南美洲 ESI 排名前 10 机构分布（图 44）

序号	是否进入ESI 前1%	机构	所属国家	被引量	发文量	篇均被引量	2020 年ESI 排名	2021 年ESI 排名	2022 年ESI 排名
1	√	圣保罗大学	巴西	609	145	4.20	222	213	202
2		智利天主教大学	智利	335	98	3.42	312	357	323
3		圣保罗联邦大学	巴西	269	46	5.85	330	430	404
4		阿雷格里港克利尼卡斯医院	巴西	268	6	44.67	510	458	407
5		卡耶塔诺·埃雷迪亚大学	秘鲁	185	26	7.12	125	596	569
6		乌贝兰迪亚联邦大学	巴西	177	13	13.62	561	654	586
7		坎皮纳斯州立大学	巴西	155	46	3.37	999	766	670
8		科拉萨奥医院	巴西	89	2	44.50	1320	1211	1049
9		米纳斯吉拉斯联邦大学	巴西	75	30	2.50	1574	1284	1197
10		智利大学	智利	67	35	1.91	1160	1390	1310

图 44　南美洲 ESI 排名前 10 机构分布

8. 中国 ESI 排名前 20 机构分布（图 45）

序号	是否进入 ESI 前 1%	机构	被引量	发文量	篇均被引量	2020 年 ESI 排名	2021 年 ESI 排名	2022 年 ESI 排名
1	√	香港大学	566	91	6.22	239	220	209
2		香港中文大学	297	45	6.60	321	428	368
3		台湾大学	284	60	4.73	395	375	383
4		北京大学	264	68	3.88	115	452	423
5		台湾大学医学院附设医院	246	49	5.02	523	502	454
6		四川大学	209	39	5.36	581	450	512
7		长庚大学	207	74	2.80	736	581	518
8		长庚纪念医院	186	48	3.88	816	614	566
9		阳明大学	167	47	3.55	781	676	623
10		中国医科大学	129	35	3.69	816	867	761
11		浙江大学	129	20	6.45	1039	902	761
12		江苏省血吸虫病防治研究所	121	2	60.50	1023	913	798
13		陆军军医大学	120	41	2.93	1009	883	806
14		中山大学	116	40	2.90	993	883	839
15		首都医科大学	107	32	3.34	1173	1008	888
16		空军军医大学	97	14	6.93	1589	1315	969
17		上海交通大学	91	34	2.68	1219	1068	1028
18		复旦大学	84	41	2.05	1383	1134	1100
19		中南大学	84	22	3.82	1436	1242	1100
20		台北医学大学	76	41	1.85	1838	1390	1181

图 45　中国 ESI 排名前 20 机构分布

五、医学教育研究期刊解析

（一）研究方法

在 JCR 数据库教育门类下的全部期刊中（包括 SCIE 收录期刊 44 种和 SSCI 收录期刊 267 种）按照纳入标准筛选出医学教育研究期刊。

纳入标准：如果某期刊近 10 年来（2011 年 1 月 1 日至 2020 年 12 月 31 日）所发表的期刊论文在 PubMed 数据库中被标引包含 "Education, Medical" [MeSH] 的比例接近或超过 50%，则认为该期刊属于医学教育研究期刊，并将其纳入分析范围。

研究方法：利用书目共现分析系统 BICOMB 统计近 10 年来全部医学教育研究期刊的高频主题词分布，用来反映该期刊的研究内容与特色主题。

（二）医学教育研究期刊总体概况（图 46）

序号	期刊名称	所属数据库	2021 年中科院期刊分区*（升级版）	影响因子（2020）	主办国家	10 年累计发文量（2011-2020）	被标引为"Education, Medical"[MeSH]的论文数量	被标引为" Education, Medical"[MeSH] 的论文比例（%）
1	Academic Medicine	SCIE	1 区	6.893	美国	4870	2515	51.64
2	Medical Education	SCIE	1 区	6.251	英国	5451	3228	59.22
3	Anatomical Sciences Education	SCIE	1 区	5.958	美国	703	365	51.92
4	Advances in Health Sciences Education	SCIE/SSCI	1 区	3.853	美国	775	383	49.42
5	Medical Teacher	SCIE	2 区	3.650	英国	3166	1907	60.23
6	Medical Education Online	SSCI	3 区	3.298	英国	596	394	66.11
7	Journal of Surgical Education	SCIE	3 区	2.891	美国	2078	1592	76.61
8	BMC Medical Education	SCIE/SSCI	3 区	2.463	英国	2837	1561	55.02
9	Teaching and Learning in Medicine	SCIE	3 区	2.414	美国	583	386	66.20
10	Academic Psychiatry	SSCI	4 区	3.293	美国	1645	972	59.09

*SCIE- 学科教育类 /SSCI- 教育学和教育研究

图 46　医学教育研究期刊总体概况

（三）医学教育学科期刊高频主题词分布

1. *Academic Medicine*（图 47）

序号	主题词	频次	百分比	A/O[1]	序号	主题词	频次	百分比	A/O[1]
1	Education, Medical	605	6.99	1.49	16	Curriculum	97	1.12	1.55
2	Students, Medical	516	5.96	1.66	17	Competency-Based Education	86	0.99	2.79
3	Education, Medical, Undergraduate	420	4.85	1.45	18	Teaching	82	0.95	0.73
4	Internship and Residency	358	4.14	0.82	19	Pediatrics	70	0.81	0.43
5	Physicians	296	3.42	2.33	20	Health Personnel	63	0.73	1.38
6	Education, Medical, Graduate	290	3.35	0.84	21	Family Practice	60	0.69	0.92
7	Schools, Medical	264	3.05	3.73	22	Health Occupations	59	0.68	3.34
8	Faculty, Medical	223	2.58	3.51	23	Research Personnel	48	0.55	5.59
9	Educational Measurement	214	2.47	1.46	24	Minority Groups	47	0.54	6.59
10	Academic Medical Centers	188	2.17	8.15	25	Patient Care Team	44	0.51	1.86
11	Internal Medicine	177	2.05	2.37	26	General Surgery	44	0.51	0.25
12	Clinical Competence	140	1.62	0.85	27	Burnout, Professional	44	0.51	1.37
13	Biomedical Research	127	1.47	2.34	28	Physicians, Primary Care	43	0.50	3.13
14	Delivery of Health Care	101	1.17	3.47	29	Problem-Based Learning	41	0.47	0.98
15	Clinical Clerkship	99	1.14	2.51	30	Staff Development	41	0.47	3.17

图 47　Academic Medicine 高频主题词分布

① A/O：A 表示相应主题词在本期刊所发表的全部论文中所占的比例；O 表示相应主题词在 PubMed 数据库中被标引为 "Education, Medical" [MeSH] 的全部期刊论文中所占的比例；A/O 用来衡量该期刊相应主题词所代表的研究内容的发表倾向程度，其值越大，表示该期刊发表关于相应主题词所代表的研究内容的比重越大，可以为医学教育研究者选择投稿期刊提供参考性意见（红色部分为 A/O 大于 5 的主题词，为重点关注内容）。

2. *Medical Education*（图 48）

序号	主题词	频次	百分比	A/O	序号	主题词	频次	百分比	A/O
1	Students, Medical	955	10.20	2.84	16	Health Occupations	76	0.81	4.05
2	Education, Medical, Undergraduate	602	6.43	1.93	17	Computer-Assisted Instruction	74	0.79	1.76
3	Education, Medical	580	6.19	1.32	18	Pediatrics	69	0.74	0.62
4	Clinical Competence	429	4.58	2.40	19	Biomedical Research	67	0.72	1.14
5	Educational Measurement	368	3.93	2.31	20	Medical Staff, Hospital	67	0.72	1.80
6	Internship and Residency	194	2.07	0.41	21	General Practice	63	0.67	1.52
7	Teaching	181	1.93	1.50	22	Stress, Psychological	61	0.65	2.71
8	Education, Medical, Graduate	151	1.61	0.40	23	Curriculum	58	0.62	0.86
9	Problem-Based Learning	148	1.58	3.31	24	Education, Medical, Continuing	57	0.61	0.37
10	Physicians	143	1.53	1.04	25	Professional Competence	57	0.61	3.81
11	Health Personnel	116	1.24	2.34	26	Competency-Based Education	53	0.57	1.63
12	Schools, Medical	115	1.23	1.50	27	Evidence-Based Medicine	48	0.51	2.55
13	Faculty, Medical	97	1.04	1.42	28	Students, Health Occupations	47	0.50	4.55
14	Internal Medicine	96	1.03	1.20	29	Family Practice	45	0.48	0.64
15	Clinical Clerkship	82	0.88	1.96	30	Students, Nursing	42	0.45	5.00

图 48　*Medical Education* 高频主题词分布

3. *Anatomical Sciences Education*（图 49）

序号	主题词	频次	百分比	A/O	序号	主题词	频次	百分比	A/O
1	Anatomy	529	26.21	33.18	16	Tissue and Organ Procurement	19	0.94	31.33
2	Education, Medical, Undergraduate	204	10.11	3.03	17	Tissue Donors	18	0.89	29.67
3	Students, Medical	153	7.58	2.11	18	Health Occupations	17	0.84	4.20
4	Teaching	120	5.95	4.61	19	Education, Professional	16	0.79	11.29
5	Dissection	63	3.12	20.80	20	Anatomists	14	0.69	34.50
6	Educational Measurement	46	2.28	1.34	21	Physical Therapy Specialty	12	0.59	9.83
7	Computer-Assisted Instruction	46	2.28	5.07	22	Faculty	11	0.55	5.00
8	Education, Medical	38	1.88	0.40	23	Education, Distance	10	0.50	1.85
9	Students	32	1.59	12.23	24	Anatomy, Regional	9	0.45	22.50
10	Histology	29	1.44	36.00	25	Anatomy, Cross-Sectional	9	0.45	45.00
11	Problem-Based Learning	28	1.39	2.90	26	Radiology	9	0.45	0.58
12	Neuroanatomy	25	1.24	31.00	27	Physiology	8	0.40	4.00
13	Curriculum	23	1.14	1.58	28	Education, Veterinary	8	0.40	13.33
14	Students, Health Occupations	21	1.04	9.45	29	Education, Medical, Graduate	8	0.40	0.10
15	Schools, Medical	21	1.04	1.27	30	Imaging, Three-Dimensional	7	0.35	11.67

图 49　*Anatomical Sciences Education* 高频主题词分布

4. *Advances in Health Sciences Education*（图 50）

序号	主题词	频次	百分比	A/O	序号	主题词	频次	百分比	A/O
1	Students, Medical	124	9.23	2.57	16	Science	15	1.12	7.00
2	Educational Measurement	102	7.59	4.46	17	Students, Health Occupations	15	1.12	10.18
3	Education, Medical	87	6.48	1.38	18	Clinical Clerkship	14	1.04	2.31
4	Education, Medical, Undergraduate	61	4.54	1.36	19	Internal Medicine	13	0.97	1.13
5	Health Occupations	44	3.28	16.40	20	School Admission Criteria	13	0.97	10.78
6	Clinical Competence	40	2.98	1.56	21	Workplace	11	0.82	10.51
7	Schools, Medical	35	2.60	3.17	22	Competency-Based Education	11	0.82	1.82
8	Problem-Based Learning	35	2.60	5.42	23	Computer-Assisted Instruction	10	0.74	1.64
9	Teaching	34	2.53	1.96	24	Cardiology	9	0.67	1.56
10	Physicians	30	2.23	1.52	25	Students, Nursing	8	0.60	6.67
11	Education, Medical, Graduate	26	1.94	0.49	26	Students	8	0.60	4.62
12	Health of Personnel	26	1.94	3.66	27	Licensure, Medical	8	0.60	6.67
13	Internship and Residency	24	1.79	0.36	28	Physical Therapy Specialty	8	0.60	10.00
14	Research	18	1.34	9.57	29	Staff Development	8	0.60	4.00
15	Faculty, Medical	18	1.34	1.84	30	Patient Care Team	8	0.60	2.22

图 50　*Advances in Health Sciences Education* 高频主题词分布

5. *Medical Teacher*（图 51）

序号	主题词	频次	百分比	A/O	序号	主题词	频次	百分比	A/O
1	Education, Medical	520	11.54	2.47	16	Health Occupations	41	0.91	4.55
2	Students, Medical	499	11.07	3.08	17	Staff Development	40	0.89	5.93
3	Education, Medical, Undergraduate	393	8.72	2.61	18	Education, Distance	34	0.75	2.78
4	Educational Measurement	259	5.75	3.38	19	Internal Medicine	33	0.73	0.85
5	Teaching	194	4.31	3.34	20	Medical Staff, Hospital	31	0.69	1.64
6	Schools, Medical	119	2.64	3.22	21	Curriculum	30	0.67	0.93
7	Clinical Competence	106	2.35	1.23	22	Computer-Assisted Instruction	29	0.64	1.42
8	Faculty, Medical	99	2.20	3.01	23	Professionalism	25	0.55	3.93
9	Internship and Residency	99	2.20	0.44	24	Pediatrics	24	0.53	0.45
10	Health Personnel	92	2.04	3.85	25	Program Evaluation	24	0.53	4.82
11	Problem-Based Learning	89	1.98	4.13	26	Professional Competence	23	0.51	3.19
12	Education, Medical, Graduate	73	1.62	0.41	27	Research	23	0.51	3.64
13	Clinical Clerkship	71	1.58	3.51	28	Education, Medical, Continuing	22	0.49	0.29
14	Physicians	63	1.40	0.95	29	Education, Professional	21	0.47	6.71
15	Competency-Based Education	48	1.07	3.06	30	Simulation Training	20	0.44	0.56

图 51　*Medical Teacher* 高频主题词分布

6. *Medical Education Online*（图 52）

序号	主题词	频次	百分比	A/O	序号	主题词	频次	百分比	A/O
1	Students, Medical	140	11.71	3.26	16	Coronavirus Infections	12	1.00	1.67
2	Education, Medical, Undergraduate	95	7.94	2.28	17	Pneumonia, Viral	12	1.00	0.83
3	Education, Medical	80	6.69	1.43	18	Biomedical Research	11	0.92	1.46
4	Internship and Residency	62	5.18	1.03	19	Education, Distance	11	0.92	3.41
5	Educational Measurement	54	4.52	2.66	20	Emergency Medicine	10	0.84	0.93
6	Schools, Medical	37	3.09	3.77	21	Health Personnel	9	0.75	1.42
7	Teaching	31	2.59	2.01	22	Research	9	0.75	5.36
8	Clinical Competence	24	2.01	1.05	23	Computer-Assisted Instruction	9	0.75	1.67
9	Faculty, Medical	23	1.92	0.63	24	Interviews as Topic	8	0.67	9.57
10	Clinical Clerkship	23	1.92	4.27	25	Staff Development	7	0.59	3.93
11	Pediatrics	22	1.84	1.55	26	Physicians	7	0.59	0.40
12	Internal Medicine	19	1.59	1.85	27	Patient-Centered Care	7	0.59	4.21
13	Problem-Based Learning	18	1.51	3.15	28	Medical Staff, Hospital	7	0.59	1.48
14	Education, Medical, Graduate	16	1.34	0.34	29	Burnout, Professional	7	0.59	1.59
15	Stress, Psychological	15	1.25	5.21	30	Social Media	7	0.59	7.38

图 52　*Medical Education Online* 高频主题词分布

7. *Journal of Surgical Education*（图 53）

序号	主题词	频次	百分比	A/O	序号	主题词	频次	百分比	A/O
1	General Surgery	762	17.48	8.57	16	Orthopedic Procedures	32	0.73	4.87
2	Education, Medical, Graduate	342	7.84	1.96	17	Faculty, Medical	32	0.73	1.00
3	Internship and Residency	323	7.41	1.47	18	Competency-Based Education	31	0.71	2.03
4	Laparoscopy	129	2.96	4.70	19	Urology	30	0.69	1.86
5	Education, Medical, Undergraduate	116	2.66	0.80	20	Personnel Selection	29	0.67	3.19
6	Simulation Training	101	2.32	58.00	21	Cholecystectomy, Laparoscopic	28	0.64	8.00
7	Specialties, Surgical	98	2.25	6.25	22	Teaching	28	0.64	0.50
8	Orthopedics	94	2.16	3.84	23	Biomedical Research	27	0.62	0.98
9	Educational Measurement	68	1.56	0.88	24	Workload	27	0.62	2.70
10	Students, Medical	54	1.24	0.35	25	Clinical Competence	27	0.62	0.32
11	Surgery, Plastic	40	0.92	2.79	26	Gynecology	27	0.62	1.38
12	Surgeons	39	0.89	1.78	27	Patient Care Team	26	0.60	2.22
13	Suture Techniques	38	0.87	7.25	28	Vascular Surgical Procedures	26	0.60	3.16
14	Clinical Clerkship	34	0.78	1.73	29	Traumatology	26	0.60	4.62
15	Education, Medical	33	0.76	0.16	30	Robotic Surgical Procedures	25	0.57	3.35

图 53　*Journal of Surgical Education* 高频主题词分布

8. BMC Medical Education（图 54）

序号	主题词	频次	百分比	A/O	序号	主题词	频次	百分比	A/O
1	Students, Medical	551	9.64	2.69	16	General Practice	52	0.91	2.07
2	Education, Medical, Undergraduate	314	5.50	1.65	17	Stress, Psychological	45	0.79	3.29
3	Clinical Competence	256	4.48	2.35	18	Pediatrics	45	0.79	0.66
4	Education, Medical	175	3.06	0.65	19	Education, Medical, Continuing	44	0.77	0.46
5	Educational Measurement	160	2.80	1.65	20	Health Occupations	42	0.74	3.70
6	Internship and Residency	116	2.03	0.40	21	Students, Health Occupations	42	0.74	6.73
7	Problem-Based Learning	93	1.63	3.40	22	Biomedical Research	42	0.74	1.17
8	Education, Medical, Graduate	91	1.59	0.40	23	Computer-Assisted Instruction	41	0.72	1.60
9	Teaching	86	1.51	1.17	24	Students, Nursing	38	0.67	7.44
10	Physicians	79	1.38	0.94	25	Physical Therapy Specialty	36	0.63	10.50
11	Health Personnel	72	1.26	2.38	26	Professional Competence	34	0.60	3.75
12	Schools, Medical	64	1.12	1.37	27	Clinical Clerkship	33	0.58	1.29
13	Internal Medicine	60	1.05	1.22	28	Evidence-Based Medicine	32	0.56	2.80
14	Faculty, Medical	55	0.96	1.32	29	Family Practice	32	0.56	0.75
15	Medical Staff, Hospital	53	0.93	2.33	30	Burnout, Professional	32	0.56	1.51

图 54　*BMC Medical Education* 高频主题词分布

9. Teaching and Learning in Medicine（图 55）

序号	主题词	频次	百分比	A/O	序号	主题词	频次	百分比	A/O
1	Students, Medical	130	13.61	3.79	16	Curriculum	12	1.26	1.75
2	Education, Medical, Undergraduate	77	8.06	2.41	17	Emergency Medicine	11	1.15	1.28
3	Educational Measurement	52	5.45	3.21	18	Physical Examination	10	1.08	7.71
4	Clinical Competence	43	4.50	2.36	19	General Surgery	9	0.94	0.46
5	Teaching	40	4.19	3.25	20	Physicians	9	0.94	0.64
6	Education, Medical	34	3.56	0.76	21	Preceptorship	9	0.94	11.75
7	Internal Medicine	31	3.25	3.78	22	Staff Development	8	0.84	5.60
8	Education, Medical, Graduate	25	2.62	0.66	23	Health Personnel	8	0.84	1.58
9	Pediatrics	20	2.09	0.84	24	Problem-Based Learning	7	0.73	1.52
10	Clinical Clerkship	20	2.09	4.64	25	Stress, Psychological	7	0.73	3.04
11	Faculty, Medical	19	1.99	2.73	26	Surveys and Questionnaires	6	0.63	7.88
12	Internship and Residency	18	1.88	0.17	27	Professional Competence	6	0.63	3.94
13	Schools, Medical	15	1.57	1.91	28	Anatomy	5	0.52	0.66
14	Competency-Based Education	13	1.36	3.89	29	Obstetrics	5	0.52	0.18
15	Family Practice	12	1.26	1.68	30	Biomedical Research	5	0.52	0.83

图 55　*Teaching and Learning in Medicine* 高频主题词分布

10. *Academic Psychiatry*（图 56）

序号	主题词	频次	百分比	A/O	序号	主题词	频次	百分比	A/O
1	Psychiatry	786	22.63	22.86	16	Psychotherapy	38	1.09	12.11
2	Internship and Residency	252	7.25	1.44	17	Educational Measurement	38	1.09	0.64
3	Students, Medical	194	5.58	1.55	18	Suicide	35	1.01	16.83
4	Curriculum	80	2.30	3.19	19	Stress, Psychological	32	0.92	3.83
5	Physicians	73	2.10	1.43	20	Mental Health Services	30	0.86	21.50
6	Mental Disorders	64	1.84	12.27	21	Depression	29	0.83	6.92
7	Education, Medical, Graduate	58	1.67	0.42	22	Biomedical Research	28	0.81	1.29
					23	Teaching	23	0.66	0.51
8	Child Psychiatry	50	1.44	24.00	24	Schools, Medical	22	0.63	0.77
9	Education, Medical	49	1.41	0.30	25	Substance-Related Disorders	22	0.63	7.88
10	Clinical Competence	47	1.35	0.71					
11	Clinical Clerkship	46	1.32	2.93	26	Neurosciences	19	0.55	13.75
12	Burnout, Professional	43	1.24	3.35	27	Fellowships and Scholarships	17	0.49	1.53
13	Education, Medical, Undergraduate	41	1.18	0.35	28	Academic Medical Centers	15	0.43	1.59
14	Adolescent Psychiatry	39	1.12	22.50	29	Forensic Psychiatry	15	0.43	21.50
15	Faculty, Medical	38	1.09	1.49	30	Cultural Competency	14	0.40	4.00

图 56 *Academic Psychiatry* 高频主题词分布

结　语

2022 年，我们迎来了"国际医学教育研究前沿报告"发布的第五个年头，通过 2001—2020 年国际医学教育研究热点和发展状态的回顾与比较和全球医学教育教学研究专题系列的引入，让这个新生而富有活力的系列报告更加具有权威性和富有特色；通过文献概览及前沿追踪的方式，让我们紧跟医学教育发展的步伐，促进国内外医学高等院校在医学教育方面的交流与合作，研究与创新，携手推动医学教育的发展。

2022 International Medical Education Research Fronts Report

（ English Version ）

Background

With the acceleration of the internationalization of medical education, current research trends call for mutual learning, timely updates of relevant concepts, understanding of present development trends, and continuous exploration for the future of medical education research and reforms. For four consecutive years, between 2018 and 2021, we have released a series of reports on international medical education fronts. We were greatly encouraged by the compelling responses that we received from our readers. For 2022, which is the fifth year of the publication of these series of frontier reports on international medical education research, we have reviewed and compared the development status and research hotspots of medical education across the world between 2001 and 2020 and performed a thematic analysis of teaching in medical education based on content from previous versions of the report. We hope that this would help medical education researchers and medical educators around the world stay up-to-date with current trends in medical education, understand the overall development trends of international medical education, and plan for the future development of medical education research.

Objectives

Based on Web of Science and PubMed databases:

(1) To comprehensively summarize and reveal the current development status and research fronts of global medical education in 2021.

(2) To review and compare the development status and research hotspots of global medical education between 2001 and 2020.

(3) To provide reference for the new round of medical education reform by analyzing the progress and trending topics of teaching in medical education at a global level.

(4) To build the essential science indicators (ESI) ranking for medical education disciplines.

(5) To use bibliometrics to analyze journals in medical education and to provide reference for medical education researchers when selecting journals for article submission.

Methods

Data collection

Existing literature in the PubMed database was retrieved using the search term: "Education, Medical [MeSH]". The PMID of retrieved articles was matched with the literature retrieved from the Web of Science database (including SCIE and SSCI), and full bibliographic records (including the reference index for each article) were downloaded.

The scope of literature

Based on the data collection, as well as the information and classification of bibliography presented in the Web of Science database, scientometric software packages HistCite and visual analysis tool CiteSpace were used to statistically analyze the following indices in the literature: number of publications per country/region, number of citations per country/region, number of publications per institution, number of citations per institution, number of publications per author, number of citations per author, number of publications per journal, and number of citations per journal.

Research fronts

1. Distribution and clustering of high frequent MeSH terms

Based on data collection, BICOMB (Bibliographic Items Co-Occurrence Matrix Builder) was used to extract the main MeSH terms from the included literature. After eliminating characteristic MeSH terms that may apply to all studies or results, high frequent MeSH terms were counted and a list of high frequent MeSH terms was generated. A clustering toolkit (gCLUTO) was used to carry out clustering analysis by importing the generated high frequent MeSH terms matrix.

2. Co-citation clustering of references

Co-citation clustering reflects the degree of aggregation among cited articles by analyzing citation relationships. Using BICOMB and gCLUTO, we extracted and ranked the cited articles and generated a co-citation matrix from the included literature for co-citation clustering.

Results

Ⅰ. Scope of literature and research fronts of medical education research

Search Strategy: Education, Medical [MeSH] OR (*Academic Medicine / Medical Education / Medical Teacher / BMC Medical Education / Journal of Surgical Education / Advances in Health Sciences Education / Teaching and Learning in Medicine / Medical Education Online / Anatomical Sciences Education / Academic Psychiatry*) [Journal].

Scope of literature

1. Countries/regions with the most publications and citations related to medical education in 2021 (Figure 1)

Ranking	Country/ Region	Number of publications	Percentage *	Ranking	Country/ Region	Number of citations	Percentage *	Average number of citations
1	USA	4026	45.53	1	USA	5247	43.63	1.30
2	UK	776	8.78	2	UK	1013	8.42	1.31
3	Canada	630	7.12	3	Canada	944	7.85	1.50
4	Australia	286	3.23	4	Netherlands	514	4.27	2.16
5	Netherlands	238	2.69	5	Australia	505	4.20	1.77
6	Germany	229	2.59	6	PRC	302	2.51	1.44
7	PRC	210	2.37	7	Germany	228	1.90	1.00
8	India	143	1.62	8	Ireland	204	1.70	2.19
9	France	127	1.44	9	Italy	199	1.65	1.67
10	Italy	119	1.35	10	India	189	1.57	1.32
11	Switzerland	103	1.16	11	France	139	1.16	1.09
12	Brazil	93	1.05	12	Switzerland	130	1.08	1.26
13	Ireland	93	1.05	13	Poland	126	1.05	4.06
14	Japan	83	0.94	14	Saudi Arabia	125	1.04	1.89
15	Singapore	83	0.94	15	Japan	122	1.01	1.47

Figure 1　Countries/regions with the most publications and citations related to medical education in 2021

---

*The unit of precentage is "%" in this book.

2. Institutions with the most publications and citations related to medical education in 2021 (Figure 2)

Ranking	Institution	Number of publications	Percentage
1	Harvard Med Sch	291	1.49
2	Univ of Calif, San Francisco	222	1.14
3	Univ of Michigan	204	1.04
4	Univ of Washington	201	1.03
5	Univ of Toronto	194	0.99
6	Stanford Univ	178	0.91
7	Mayo Clin	155	0.79
8	Univ of Penn	149	0.76
9	Vanderbilt Univ	135	0.69
10	Massachusetts Gen Hosp	126	0.64
11	Johns Hopkins Univ	124	0.63
12	Northwestern Univ	116	0.59
13	Emory Univ	113	0.58
14	Univ of N Carolina	113	0.58
15	Ohio State Univ	109	0.57

Ranking	Institution	Number of citations	Percentage	Average number of citations
1	Harvard Med Sch	448	1.57	1.54
2	Univ of Calif, San Francisco	399	1.40	1.80
3	Univ of Michigan	371	1.30	1.82
4	Univ of Washington	370	1.30	1.84
5	Univ of Toronto	352	1.24	1.81
6	Stanford Univ	299	1.05	1.68
7	Univ of Penn	285	1.00	1.91
8	Mayo Clin	268	0.94	1.73
9	Maastricht Univ	227	0.80	2.64
10	Univ of N Carolina	227	0.80	2.01
11	Vanderbilt Univ	218	0.77	1.61
12	Massachusetts Gen Hosp	201	0.71	1.60
13	Northwestern Univ	194	0.68	1.67
14	Univ of British Columbia	172	0.60	1.83
15	Univ of Illinois	172	0.60	2.57

Figure 2　Institutions with the most publications and citations related to medical education in 2021

3. Authors with the most publications and citations related to medical education in 2021 (Figure 3)

Ranking	Author with the most publications	Institution	Number of publications
1	Hauer, Karen E.	Univ of Calif, San Francisco	23
2	Park, Yoon Soo	Harvard Med Sch	23
3	Hammoud, Maya M.	Univ of Michigan	22
4	Schumacher, Daniel J.	Univ of Cincinnati	20
5	Santen, Sally A.	Virginia Commonwealth Univ	19
6	Ten Cate, Olle	Univ of Med Ctr Utrecht	19
7	Drolet, Brain C.	Vanderbilt Univ	17
8	O'Sullivan, Patricia S.	Univ of Calif, San Francisco	16
9	Teunissen, Pim W.	Maastricht Univ	16
10	Varpio, Lara	Uniformed Serv Univ of the Hlth Sci	15
11	Cleland, Jennifer	Nanyang Technol Univ	14
12	Driessen, Erik W.	Maastricht Univ	14
13	George, Brian C.	Univ of Michigan	14
14	Ross, Shelley	Univ of Alberta	13
15	Elkbuli, Adel	Kendall Reg Med Ctr	13

Ranking	Author with the most citations	Institution	Number of citations	Average number of citations
1	Varpio, Lara	Uniformed Serv Univ of the Hlth Sci	72	4.80
2	Ten Cate, Olle	Univ of Med Ctr Utrecht	63	3.32
3	Asaad, Malke	Univ of Texas MD Anderson Canc Ctr	61	5.55
4	Dumont, Aaron S.	Tulane Univ	60	15
5	Teunissen, Pim W.	Maastricht Univ	59	3.69
6	Aziz, Hassan	Univ of Southern Calif	57	28.50
7	Iwanaga, Joe	Tulane Univ	57	28.50
8	Sullivan, Maura E.	Univ of Southern Calif	57	19.00
9	Tubbs, R. Shane	Tulane Univ	57	14.25
10	Genyk, Yuri	Univ of Southern Calif	56	56
11	Remulla, Daphne	Univ of Southern Calif	56	56
12	Sheikh, Mohd Raashid	Univ of Southern Calif	56	56
13	Sher, Linda	Univ of Southern Calif	56	56
14	James, Tayler	Univ of Southern Calif	56	56
15	Loukas, Marios	Univ of Warmia & Mazury	54	54

Figure 3　Authors with the most publications and citations related to medical education in 2021

Note: All authors were considered equally, without distinguishing between first author, corresponding author, or co-author.

Research fronts

1. Highest frequent MeSH terms from publications in medical education in 2021 (Figure 4)

Ranking	MeSH Term	Frequency	Percentage	Ranking	MeSH Term	Frequency	Percentage
1	Internship and Residency	3220	13.39	21	Surgery, Plastic	161	0.67
2	Students, Medical	1547	6.43	22	Psychiatry	149	0.62
3	COVID-19	1267	5.27	23	Schools, Medical	139	0.58
4	Education, Medical	1226	5.10	24	Education, Medical, Continuing	133	0.55
5	Education, Medical, Undergraduate	947	3.94	25	Pediatrics	120	0.50
6	Education, Medical, Graduate	533	2.22	26	Learning	120	0.50
7	Clinical Competence	432	1.80	27	Orthopedics	113	0.47
8	Physicians	387	1.61	28	Emergency Medicine	111	0.46
9	General Surgery	352	1.46	29	Dermatology	110	0.46
10	Education, Distance	295	1.23	30	Teaching Rounds	109	0.45
11	Curriculum	292	1.21	31	Ophthalmology	109	0.45
12	Surgeons	268	1.11	32	Faculty, Medical	105	0.44
13	Educational Measurement	233	0.97	33	Obstetrics	100	0.42
14	Simulation Training	201	0.84	34	Gynecology	100	0.42
15	Anatomy	183	0.76	35	Medicine	100	0.42
16	Radiology	174	0.72	36	Otolaryngology	100	0.42
17	Pandemics	173	0.72	37	Urology	99	0.41
18	Fellowships and Scholarships	165	0.69	38	Biomedical Research	98	0.41
19	Clinical Clerkship	164	0.68	39	Personnel Selection	95	0.40
20	Burnout, Professional	163	0.68	40	Neurosurgery	95	0.40

Figure 4　Highest frequent MeSH terms from publications in medical education in 2021

2. Highest frequent MeSH terms clustering of publications in medical education in 2021 (Figure 5)

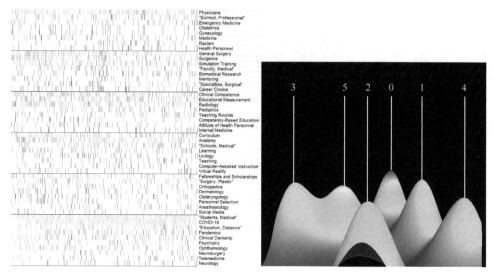

Figure 5   Highest frequent MeSH terms clustering of publications in medical education in 2021

Note: The numbers in the right figure indicate the theme categories formed by the highest frequent MeSH terms clustering of publications.

Through high frequent MeSH terms clustering, six major themes about medical education in 2021 have emerged:

(1) Research on professional practice environment and its influencing factors among health professionals.

(2) Research on the professional development of faculty in medical schools.

(3) Research on teaching and evaluation based on clinical competence.

(4) Application of digital information technology in medical teaching.

(5) The role of social media in the allocation of health human resources under the influence of the COVID-19 pandemic.

(6) Research on the reform of medical teaching models and methods under the influence of the COVID-19 pandemic

Special topic: Development and applications of medical education models

In recent years, global medical education has undergone key changes. The third-generation wave of medical education reform that began in 2010 and the current COVID-19 pandemic have prompted a rethinking of medical education. In such a historical period, medical education models are undergoing new rounds of global changes, and related research is gradually been carried out.

1. Types of medical education models

Medical education models are the products of a combination of specific time periods and backgrounds, specific learners, learning content, and learning environments, including educational goals, educational content, and training pathways, which occur alongside the development of medicine and the transformation of medical models. During the whole development process, medical education models have undergone three important phases of changes and upgrades, namely the empirical medical education model, the scientific medical education model, and the human-centered medical education model (Figure 6). Among them, the scientific medical education model is a general term for medical education models from the 18th century to the end of the 20th century, which can be further subdivided into two development stages: discipline-based medical education model and problem-based medical education model.

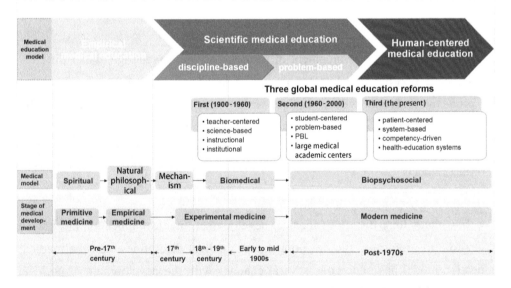

Figure 6   Schematic diagram of the evolution of medical education models

The evolution of medical education models is inseparable from the specific time era, breakthroughs in the understanding of medicine, and changes in social needs. The specific medical development stage determines the medical model at that time. The medical model of the time, combined with the learners, learning content, and learning environment of the specific time era, determines the corresponding medical education model.

As shown in Figure 6, the spiritual and natural philosophical medical model, formed under the background of primitive medicine and empirical medicine, determined the educational model for empirical medicine of its time. Entrance into the period of experimental medicine also opened the door for scientific medical education model. During this period, the world experienced the first and second generational waves of medical education reforms. Particularly, the second generation of global medical education reform became a watershed moment in the transition between discipline-based medical education and problem-based medical education. The 1970s saw the initial development of what is known as modern medicine and opened the way for the biopsychosocial medical model. At present, since the beginning of the 21st century, the human-centered medical education model came into practice alongside the third-generation wave of competency-oriented medical education reform. This current human-centered medical education model will continue to mature and develop long into the future.

2. Applications of medical education models

(1) Medical education models in various countries

From the budding development of medicine to the present age, under different medical education models, different countries and schools have emerged and become the pioneer representatives of various time periods. Table 1 summarizes health professional training goals, training pathways, teaching models, teaching methods, and learning theories of medical education under different countries and different medical education models.

(2) Exploration of China's medical education model

In China's long history of medical development, medical education has played a key role in promoting the development of medical disciplines, and the medical education model has undergone several changes with the development of politics, economy, and society. From primarily taking traditional Chinese medicine to the budding of Western medicine, China has strived to explore medical education models based on overall national conditions in each historical development period and has made brilliant achievements.

Table 1   Medical education models and countries/institutions of practice

Medical education model		Period	Representative countries and institutions	Professional outcome	Training pathways	Teaching models	Teaching methods
Empirical medical education model		pre-1900	The Schola Medica Salernitana, Italy; China	Witch doctor; missionary; Traditional Chinese doctor	Apprenticeship; scholastic medical education	Master and apprentice; authoritative medical writings and religious/philosophical knowledge	Word of mouth; practical teaching
Scientific medical education model	Discipline-based medical education model	1900 to 1960	Johns Hopkins University School of Medicine, USA; Charité Medical University, Germany; Faculty of Medicine, University of Tokyo, Japan	Applicable specialists	USA: 3-year system changed to (2+2)-year system, and then changed to 5-year system; Germany: (2+1)-year system; Japan: (3+3)-year system to (3+4)-year system	The classical medical curriculum model: a discipline-based basic-clinical curriculum system	Closed teaching, indoctrination teaching methods; bedside teaching
	Problem-based medical education model	1960 to 2000	McMaster University School of Medicine, Canada; University of Dundee School of Medicine, UK; Tokyo Medical University, Japan	Comprehensively developed professionals	Canada, USA: (4+4)-year system (4 years undergraduate degree + 4 years medical school) UK: 7-year system Japan: (2+4+1)-year system	Integrated curriculum	Problem-based learning (PBL); standardized patients
Human-centered medical education model		2000-present	Harvard Medical School, USA; University of Oxford Medical School, UK	Medical professionals equipped with excellence and competency	USA: (4+4)-year system (see above) UK: 6-year system	Competency-oriented, horizontal integration between courses and vertical integration between course levels	Diversified teaching methods, such as case-based collaborative learning

During the period of the empirical medical education model, the Chinese medical education curriculum experienced numerous changes alongside the sociopolitical changes of the country, but all were based on the classics of traditional Chinese medicine (TCM). TCM medical education has experienced various stages of germination, development, and peaking. After the Communist Party of China (CPC) was established, medical schools were actively established in many revolutionary bases to learn the Soviet model and they vigorously developed medical education. Higher medical education led by the CPC was closely linked with the development of the nation, forming a relatively independent and complete medical education system and laying the foundation for the establishment and development of medical education in the New China.

After the founding of the People's Republic of China, the CPC and the people's government formulated China's education policy and health care guidelines and clarified that education, health, and other departments of medical education would gradually form China's unique higher medical education system in accordance with China's development directions and missions. As such, China officially stepped into the era of the scientific medical education model. Since the National Medical Education Reform Work Conference in 2011, China has carried out a series of profound changes in its medical education training system, which has laid a solid foundation for the development of the human-centered medical education model.

China has a sizable supply of medical education resources, and the scale of medical education in China ranks among the top in the world. However, from the perspective of social demands, China still has a large gap to fill for top-notch innovative medical talents; medical education resources are still relatively low in terms of ratios and demands; there is a continued need for the increase in number of primary care physicians; and there is a strong need for the reform of the public health system, among other practical problems. In this context, China urgently needs to explore a practical way for human-centered medical education that suits the present needs of the country.

Human development and the progression of society have determined the birth and evolution of medical education models. Since the new era, China's medical education model has been in a critical period of transformation. Through new requirements for professional training goals, the construction of a new training system, and the in-depth integration of multiple disciplines, China has optimized the supply and demand relationship between medical education and the health care system, thereby establishing a new medical education model to promote the reform and innovation of medical education.

Recommended reading:

[1] Wen D L, Ding N. Higher medical education led by the Communist Party of China: developments, achievements and implications[J]. China Higher Education Research, 2021, (8): 17-25.

[2] Zhao T L, Cao Y F, Liu L, et al. The evolution of medical education model and its motivation[J]. Health Vocational Education, 2011, 29(21): 5-7.

[3] Jin Z J. Talking about the model of medicine and curriculum of medical education[J]. Health Vocational Education, 2003, 21(12): 6-9.

[4] Hu J P, Zhai S Q, Wang J. Formation and development of the theoretical system for traditional Chinese medicine[J]. Clinical Journal of Traditional Chinese Medicine, 2015, 27(8): 1051-1054.

[5] Gao A G. Analyzing and thinking of Chinese medical educational reform and developing in 21st century[D]. The Fourth Military Medical University, 2001.

[6] Guo Y S. A preliminary study on the medical education model[J]. Medical Education (China), 1989, 70(4): 1-3.

[7] Sun B Z. Medical curriculum models reform centenary in the world and for reference[J]. Chinese Journal of Medical Education, 2012, 32(1): 1-7.

[8] Frenk J, Chen L, Bhutta ZA, et al. Health professionals for a new century: transforming education to strengthen health systems in an interdependent world[J]. Lancet, 2010, 376(9756): 1923-1958.

[9] Wijnen-Meijer M, Burdick W, Alofs L, et al. Stages and transitions in medical education around the world: clarifying structures and terminology[J]. Medical Teacher, 2013, 35(4): 7.

[10] Li M L, Ding R X, Zhang Y, et al. From cognitive sciences to learning sciences: the past, the present and the future[J]. Tsinghua Journal of Education, 2018, 39(4): 29-39.

Ⅱ. Scope of literature and research hotspots of medical education research between 2001 and 2020

Search Strategy: "Education, Medical" [MeSH] OR (*Academic Medicine/Medical Education/Medical Teacher/BMC Medical Education/Journal of Surgical Education/ Advances in Health Sciences Education/Teaching and Learning in Medicine/Medical*

Education Online/Anatomical Sciences Education/Academic Psychiatry) [Journal].

　　Time range: 2001-01-01—2020-12-31.

　　Document Type: Article.

Scope of literature

1. Countries/regions with the most publications and citations related to medical education between 2001 and 2005 (Figure 7)

Ranking	Country/Region	Number of publications	Percentage	Ranking	Country/Region	Number of citations	Percentage	Average number of citations
1	USA	4131	51.38	1	USA	142 730	52.88	34.55
2	UK	1177	14.64	2	UK	41 934	15.54	35.63
3	Canada	674	8.38	3	Canada	28 412	10.53	42.15
4	Australia	332	4.13	4	Netherlands	10 941	4.05	50.42
5	Netherlands	217	2.70	5	Australia	9266	3.43	27.91
6	Germany	203	2.52	6	Germany	3836	1.42	18.90
7	France	96	1.19	7	Israel	2523	0.93	35.04
8	Italy	76	0.95	8	Sweden	2392	0.89	39.21
9	Israel	72	0.90	9	Denmark	2197	0.81	46.74
10	New Zealand	62	0.77	10	New Zealand	2064	0.76	33.29
11	Sweden	61	0.76	11	Switzerland	1847	0.68	30.78
12	Switzerland	60	0.75	12	Italy	1764	0.65	23.21
13	PRC	58	0.72	13	Brazil	1576	0.58	32.83
14	Turkey	54	0.67	14	Belgium	1533	0.57	41.43
15	Spain	53	0.66	15	Norway	1519	0.56	39.97

Figure 7　Countries/regions with the most publications and citations related to medical education between 2001 and 2005

2. Countries/regions with the most publications and citations related to medical education between 2006 and 2010 (Figure 8)

Ranking	Country/Region	Number of publications	Percentage	Ranking	Country/Region	Number of citations	Percentage	Average number of citations
1	USA	6159	44.67	1	USA	188 898	46.70	30.67
2	UK	1476	10.71	2	Canada	44 086	10.90	39.43
3	Canada	1118	8.11	3	UK	42 792	10.58	28.99
4	Australia	571	4.14	4	Netherlands	18 580	4.59	41.75
5	Germany	520	3.77	5	Australia	15 553	3.84	27.24
6	Netherlands	445	3.23	6	Germany	11 150	2.76	21.44
7	France	207	1.50	7	Italy	4990	1.23	29.70
8	PRC	170	1.23	8	France	4591	1.13	22.18
9	Italy	168	1.22	9	Spain	4118	1.02	25.74
10	Spain	160	1.16	10	Sweden	4060	1.00	32.74
11	Japan	136	0.99	11	Switzerland	4012	0.99	30.63
12	Brazil	131	0.95	12	Japan	3812	0.94	28.03
13	Switzerland	131	0.95	13	PRC	3518	0.87	20.69
14	Sweden	124	0.90	14	Denmark	2994	0.74	35.64
15	Israel	97	0.71	15	Belgium	2812	0.70	30.24

Figure 8　Countries/regions with the most publications and citations related to medical education between 2006 and 2010

3. Countries/regions with the most publications and citations related to medical education between 2011 and 2015 (Figure 9)

Ranking	Country/Region	Number of publications	Percentage	Ranking	Country/Region	Number of citations	Percentage	Average number of citations
1	USA	7935	42.41	1	USA	174 489	42.24	21.99
2	Canada	1724	9.21	2	Canada	44 501	10.77	25.81
3	UK	1683	9.00	3	UK	44 017	10.65	26.15
4	Australia	869	4.64	4	Netherlands	21 253	5.14	29.85
5	Germany	718	3.84	5	Australia	18 894	4.57	21.74
6	Netherlands	712	3.81	6	Germany	12 488	3.02	17.39
7	PRC	308	1.65	7	France	5814	1.41	19.32
8	France	301	1.61	8	Switzerland	5780	1.40	26.15
9	Switzerland	221	1.18	9	Italy	5619	1.36	26.50
10	Italy	212	1.13	10	Belgium	4935	1.19	31.43
11	Spain	197	1.13	11	PRC	4725	1.14	15.34
12	Brazil	188	1.05	12	Denmark	4269	1.03	25.11
13	Japan	180	1.00	13	Spain	3700	0.90	18.78
14	Saudi Arabia	173	0.94	14	Sweden	3622	0.88	21.56
15	Denmark	170	0.91	15	Brazil	3287	0.80	17.48

Figure 9　Countries/regions with the most publications and citations related to medical education between 2011 and 2015

4. Countries/regions with the most publications and citations related to medical education between 2016 and 2020 (Figure 10)

Ranking	Country/Region	Number of publications	Percentage	Ranking	Country/Region	Number of citations	Percentage	Average number of citations
1	USA	9884	41.81	1	USA	94 268	41.83	9.54
2	Canada	2029	8.58	2	Canada	22 249	9.87	10.97
3	UK	1653	6.99	3	UK	16 613	7.37	10.05
4	Australia	1096	4.64	4	Australia	11 208	4.97	10.23
5	Netherlands	921	3.90	5	Netherlands	10 606	4.71	11.52
6	Germany	882	3.73	6	Germany	7711	3.42	8.74
7	PRC	556	2.35	7	PRC	4747	2.11	8.54
8	France	403	1.70	8	Italy	3490	1.55	11.71
9	Italy	298	1.26	9	France	3058	1.36	7.59
10	Spain	296	1.25	10	Spain	2705	1.20	9.14
11	Switzerland	290	1.23	11	Switzerland	2699	1.20	9.31
12	Brazil	279	1.18	12	Denmark	2454	1.09	11.47
13	Japan	259	1.10	13	Ireland	2317	1.03	10.21
14	India	241	1.02	14	Sweden	2187	0.97	10.94
15	Ireland	227	0.96	15	Belgium	2169	0.96	13.64

Figure 10　Countries/regions with the most publications and citations related to medical education between 2016 and 2020

5. Ranking analysis of countries/regions with the most publications and citations related to medical education between 2001 and 2020 (Figure 11)

Country/Region	Publication ranking				Country/Region	Citation ranking			
	2001—2005	2006—2010	2011—2015	2016—2020		2001—2005	2006—2010	2011—2015	2016—2020
USA	1	1	1	1	USA	1	1	1	1
Canada	3	3	2	2	Canada	3	2	2	2
UK	2	2	3	3	UK	2	3	3	3
Australia	4	4	4	4	Australia	5	5	5	4
Netherlands	5	6	6	5	Netherlands	4	4	4	5
Germany	6	5	5	6	Germany	6	6	6	6
PRC	13	8	7	7	PRC	20	13	11	7
France	7	7	8	8	Italy	12	7	9	8
Italy	8	9	10	9	France	16	8	7	9
Spain	15	10	11	10	Spain	18	9	13	10
Switzerland	12	12	9	11	Switzerland	11	11	8	11
Brazil	16	12	12	12	Denmark	9	14	12	12
Japan	22	11	13	13	Ireland	21	16	17	13
India	26	20	19	14	Sweden	8	10	14	14
Ireland	25	19	17	15	Belgium	14	15	10	15

Figure 11 Ranking analysis of countries/regions with the most publications and citations related to medical education between 2001 and 2020

6. Institutions with the most publications and citations related to medical education between 2001 and 2005 (Figure 12)

Ranking	Institution	Number of publications	Percentage
1	Univ of Toronto	213	1.46
2	Harvard Univ	207	1.42
3	Univ of Texas	199	1.37
4	Univ of Washington	190	1.30
5	Univ of Calif, San Francisco	156	1.07
6	Univ of Michigan	127	0.87
7	Univ of Penn	105	0.72
8	Univ of Pittsburgh	101	0.69
9	Yale Univ	99	0.68
10	Univ of N Carolina	91	0.62
11	Univ of Calif, Los Angeles	90	0.62
12	Johns Hopkins Univ	87	0.60
13	Northwestern Univ	83	0.57
14	McMaster Univ	82	0.56
15	Univ of Illinois	81	0.56

Ranking	Institution	Number of citations	Percentage	Average number of citations
1	Harvard Univ	11 670	2.24	56.38
2	Univ of Washington	9772	1.88	51.43
3	Univ of Toronto	9084	1.75	42.65
4	Univ of Texas	6439	1.24	32.36
5	Yale Univ	6174	1.19	62.36
6	Univ of Calif, San Francisco	6130	1.18	39.29
7	Northwestern Univ	5454	1.05	65.71
8	Univ of Penn	5253	1.01	50.03
9	Univ of Michigan	5073	0.97	39.94
10	McMaster Univ	5063	0.97	61.74
11	Duke Univ	4694	0.90	67.06
12	Brigham & Women's Hosp	4448	0.85	98.84
13	Johns Hopkins Univ	3654	0.70	42.00
14	Univ of Maastricht	3634	0.70	66.07
15	Emory Univ	3527	0.68	54.26

Figure 12 Institutions with the most publications and citations related to medical education between 2001 and 2005

7. Institutions with the most publications and citations related to medical education between 2006 and 2010 (Figure 13)

Ranking	Institution	Number of publications	Percentage
1	Harvard Univ	362	1.42
2	Univ of Toronto	338	1.33
3	Univ of Calif, San Francisco	272	1.07
4	Univ of Washington	271	1.07
5	Mayo Clin	218	0.86
6	Univ of Michigan	188	0.74
7	Johns Hopkins Univ	186	0.73
8	Univ of Penn	171	0.67
9	Univ of Pittsburgh	158	0.62
10	Yale Univ	152	0.60
11	Univ of Calif, Los Angeles	143	0.56
12	Univ of British Columbia	135	0.53
13	Duke Univ	133	0.52
14	McMaster Univ	129	0.51
15	Northwestern Univ	125	0.49

Ranking	Institution	Number of citations	Percentage	Average number of citations
1	Harvard Univ	15 320	1.88	42.32
2	Univ of Toronto	14 438	1.78	42.72
3	Univ of Calif, San Francisco	11 032	1.36	40.56
4	Mayo Clin	10 368	1.28	47.56
5	Univ of Washington	10 367	1.28	38.25
6	Northwestern Univ	8818	1.08	70.54
7	McMaster Univ	7901	0.97	61.25
8	Univ of Penn	6698	0.82	39.17
9	Johns Hopkins Univ	6652	0.82	35.76
10	Yale Univ	6544	0.80	43.05
11	Univ of Michigan	6526	0.80	34.71
12	Duke Univ	5843	0.72	43.93
13	Univ of British Columbia	5438	0.67	40.28
14	Brigham & Women's Hosp	5421	0.67	58.29
15	Univ of Pittsburgh	5261	0.65	33.30

Figure 13　Institutions with the most publications and citations related to medical education between 2006 and 2010

8. Institutions with the most publications and citations related to medical education between 2011 and 2015 (Figure 14)

Ranking	Institution	Number of publications	Percentage
1	Univ of Toronto	531	1.37
2	Harvard Univ	520	1.34
3	Univ of Washington	435	1.12
4	Univ of Calif, San Francisco	359	0.93
5	Mayo Clin	323	0.84
6	Maastricht Univ	271	0.70
7	Univ of Michigan	270	0.70
8	Univ of Penn	245	0.63
9	Univ of British Columbia	236	0.61
10	Northwestern Univ	229	0.59
11	Johns Hopkins Univ	229	0.59
12	Stanford Univ	225	0.58
13	Yale Univ	213	0.55
14	Duke Univ	208	0.54
15	Massachusetts Gen Hosp	208	0.54

Ranking	Institution	Number of citations	Percentage	Average number of citations
1	Univ of Toronto	14 702	1.60	27.69
2	Harvard Univ	14 480	1.58	27.85
3	Mayo Clin	13 795	1.51	42.71
4	Univ of Calif, San Francisco	12 637	1.38	35.20
5	Univ of Washington	12 629	1.38	29.03
6	Maastricht Univ	9730	1.06	35.90
7	Univ of Michigan	8207	0.90	30.40
8	Northwestern Univ	7675	0.84	33.52
9	Yale Univ	7412	0.81	34.80
10	Univ of British Columbia	7317	0.80	31.00
11	Stanford Univ	6415	0.70	28.51
12	Univ of Penn	6231	0.68	25.43
13	Massachusetts Gen Hosp	6016	0.66	28.92
14	Brigham & Women's Hosp	5763	0.63	31.49
15	Univ of Dundee	5605	0.61	59.00

Figure 14　Institutions with the most publications and citations related to medical education between 2011 and 2015

9. Institutions with the most publications and citations related to medical education between 2016 and 2020 (Figure 15)

Ranking	Institution	Number of publications	Percentage
1	Harvard Med Sch	642	1.18
2	Univ of Toronto	627	1.15
3	Univ of Washington	559	1.03
4	Univ of Calif, San Francisco	506	0.93
5	Univ of Michigan	463	0.85
6	Mayo Clin	400	0.73
7	Univ of Penn	383	0.70
8	Stanford Univ	371	0.68
9	Maastricht Univ	342	0.63
10	Northwestern Univ	319	0.59
11	Johns Hopkins Univ	305	0.56
12	Univ of Ottawa	299	0.55
13	Univ of Colorado	287	0.53
14	Univ of British Columbia	273	0.50
15	Massachusetts Gen Hosp	263	0.48

Ranking	Institution	Number of citations	Percentage	Average number of citations
1	Harvard Med Sch	7023	1.28	10.94
2	Univ of Toronto	6911	1.26	11.02
3	Univ of Calif, San Francisco	6698	1.22	13.24
4	Univ of Washington	6651	1.21	11.90
5	Mayo Clin	5420	0.99	13.55
6	Univ of Michigan	5142	0.94	11.11
7	Univ of Penn	5110	0.93	13.34
8	Stanford Univ	4565	0.83	12.30
9	Northwestern Univ	4374	0.80	13.71
10	Univ of Ottawa	4209	0.77	14.08
11	Maastricht Univ	4107	0.75	12.01
12	McGill Univ	3610	0.66	14.50
13	Johns Hopkins Univ	3496	0.64	11.46
14	Univ of Minnesota	3413	0.62	14.46
15	Massachusetts Gen Hosp	3266	0.59	12.42

Figure 15　Institutions with the most publications and citations related to medical education between 2016 and 2020

10. Ranking analysis of institutions with the most publications and citations related to medical education between 2001 and 2020 (Figure 16)

Institution	Publication ranking			
	2001—2005	2006—2010	2011—2015	2016—2020
Harvard Med Sch	444	655	1101	1
Univ of Toronto	1	2	1	2
Univ of Washington	4	4	3	3
Univ of Calif, San Francisco	5	3	4	4
Univ of Michigan	6	6	7	5
Mayo Clin	40	5	5	6
Univ of Penn	7	8	8	7
Stanford Univ	19	19	12	8
Maastricht Univ	37	25	6	9
Northwestern Univ	13	15	10	10
Johns Hopkins Univ	12	7	10	11
Univ of Ottawa	75	49	23	12
Univ of Colorado	17	28	27	13
Univ of British Columbia	48	12	9	14
Massachusetts Gen Hosp	24	23	14	15
Harvard Univ	2	1	2	70

Institution	Citation ranking			
	2001—2005	2006—2010	2011—2015	2016—2020
Harvard Med Sch	987	1266	293	1
Univ of Toronto	3	2	1	2
Univ of Calif, San Francisco	6	3	4	3
Univ of Washington	2	5	5	4
Mayo Clin	41	4	3	5
Univ of Michigan	9	11	7	6
Univ of Penn	8	8	12	7
Stanford Univ	20	17	11	8
Northwestern Univ	7	6	8	9
Univ of Ottawa	85	28	22	10
Maastricht Univ	33	21	6	11
McGill Univ	17	19	19	12
Johns Hopkins Univ	13	9	16	13
Univ of Minnesota	55	22	29	14
Massachusetts Gen Hosp	23	16	13	15
Harvard Univ	1	1	2	42

Figure 16　Ranking analysis of institutions with the most publications and citations related to medical education between 2001 and 2020

11. Authors with the most publications and citations related to medical education between 2001 and 2005 (Figure 17)

Ranking	Author with the most publications	Institution	Number of publications
1	van der Vleuten, Cees P. M.	Maastricht Univ	63
2	Regehr, Glenn	Univ of Toronto	39
3	Scherpbier, Albert J. J. A.	Maastricht Univ	36
4	Boulet, John R.	Educational Commission for Foreign Medical Graduates	30
5	Mohammadreza Hojat	Thomas Jefferson Univ	21
6	Geoffrey R. Norman	McMaster Univ	21
7	Cees van der Vleuten	Maastricht Univ	20
8	Diana H.J.M. Dolmans	Maastricht Univ	19
9	Judy A. Shea	Univ of Penn	19
10	Darzi, Ara	Imperial Coll London	18
11	Joseph S. Gonnella	Thomas Jefferson Univ	18
12	Scott M. Wright	Johns Hopkins Univ	18
13	Tim Dornan	Univ of Manchester	17
14	Ronald M. Harden	Univ of Dundee	17
15	Clarence D. Kreiter	Univ of Iowa	17

Ranking	Author with the most citations	Institution	Number of citations	Average number of citations
1	van der Vleuten, Cees P. M.	Maastricht Univ	3952	62.73
2	Regehr, Glenn	Univ of Toronto	2891	74.13
3	McGaghie, William C.	Northwestern Univ	2484	177.43
4	A. G. Gallagher	Emory Univ	2432	304.00
5	John W. Cronin	Brigham & Women's Hosp	2402	800.67
6	Charles A. Czeisler	Brigham & Women's Hosp	2402	800.67
7	R. M. Satava	Univ of Washington	2327	387.83
8	Kevin W. Eva	McMaster Univ	2243	160.21
9	S. Barry Issenberg	Univ of Miami	2178	272.25
10	Mohammadreza Hojat	Thomas Jefferson Univ	2159	102.81
11	David Lee Gordon	Univ of Miami	2114	352.33
12	Emil R. Petrusa	Duke Univ	2055	342.50
13	Joel T. Katz	Brigham & Women's Hosp	1909	477.25
14	Ross J. Scalese	Univ of Miami	1898	1898.00
15	William T. Branch Jr	Emory Univ	1891	145.46

Figure 17 Authors with the most publications and citations related to medical education between 2001 and 2005

12. Authors with the most publications and citations related to medical education between 2006 and 2010 (Figure 18)

Ranking	Author with the most publications	Institution	Number of publications
1	van der Vleuten, Cees P. M.	Maastricht Univ	50
2	Scherpbier, Albert J. J. A.	Maastricht Univ	39
3	Durning, Steven J.	Uniformed Serv Univ of the Hlth Sci	32
4	Cook, David A.	Mayo Clin	31
5	Darzi, Ara	Imperial Coll London	31
6	Boulet, John R.	Fdn Adv Int Med Educ & Res	28
7	Dubrowski, Adam	Univ of Toronto	28
8	Muijtjens, Arno M. M.	Maastricht Univ	28
9	Eva, Kevin W.	McMaster Univ	26
10	Beckman, Thomas J.	Mayo Clin	25
11	McGaghie, William C.	Northwestern Univ	25
12	Regehr, Glenn	Univ of British Columbia	25
13	Aggarwal, Rajesh	Imperial Coll London	24
14	Cohen-Schotanus, Janke	Univ of Groningen	24
15	Holmboe, Eric S.	Amer Board Internal Med	24

Ranking	Author with the most citations	Institution	Number of citations	Average number of citations
1	McGaghie, William C.	Northwestern Univ	4292	171.68
2	Wayne, Diane B.	Northwestern Univ	2639	138.89
3	Shanafelt, Tait D.	Mayo Clin	2467	224.27
4	Frank, Jason R.	Univ of Ottawa	2434	270.44
5	Norman, Geoff	McMaster Univ	2414	142.00
6	Sloan, Jeff A.	Mayo Clin	2410	301.25
7	Ten Cate, Olle	Univ of Med Ctr Utrecht	2325	166.07
8	West, Colin P.	Mayo Clin	2173	127.82
9	Cook, David A.	Mayo Clin	2136	68.90
10	van der Vleuten, Cees P. M.	Maastricht Univ	2056	41.12
11	Darzi, Ara	Imperial Coll London	2005	64.68
12	Barsuk, Jeffrey H.	Northwestern Univ	1954	217.11
13	Regehr, Glenn	Univ of British Columbia	1853	74.12
14	Aggarwal, Rajesh	Imperial Coll London	1852	77.17
15	Holmboe, Eric S.	Amer Board Internal Med	1755	73.13

Figure 18 Authors with the most publications and citations related to medical education between 2006 and 2010

13. Authors with the most publications and citations related to medical education between 2011 and 2015 (Figure 19)

Ranking	Author with the most publicatins	Institution	Number of publications
1	van der Vleuten, Cees P. M.	Maastricht Univ	85
2	Durning, Steven J.	Uniformed Serv Univ of the Hlth Sci	61
3	van der Vleuten, Cees	Maastricht Univ	47
4	Artino, Anthony R., Jr.	Uniformed Serv Univ of the Hlth Sci	46
5	Scherpbier, Albert J. J. A.	Maastricht Univ	46
6	Darzi, Ara	Imperial Coll London	41
7	Aggarwal, Rajesh	McGill Univ	40
8	Dornan, Tim	Maastricht Univ	36
9	Ringsted, Charlotte	Univ of Toronto	35
10	Regehr, Glenn	Univ of British Columbia	33
11	Cook, David A.	Mayo Clin	32
12	Scheele, Fedde	Vrije Univ Amsterdam	30
13	Holmboe, Eric S.	Accreditat Council Grad Med Educ	29
14	Lingard, Lorelei	Univ of Western Ontario	29
15	Ahmed, Kamran	King's Coll London	28

Ranking	Author with the most citations	Institution	Number of citations	Average number of citations
1	Cook, David A.	Mayo Clin	4188	130.88
2	van der Vleuten, Cees P. M.	Maastricht Univ	3715	43.71
3	Reed, Darcy A.	Mayo Clin	3348	152.18
4	Guthrie, Bruce	Univ of Dundee	3102	1034.00
5	Norbury, Michael	Univ of Dundee	3095	1547.50
6	Barnett, Karen	Univ of Dundee	3075	3075.00
7	Mercer, Stewart W.	Univ of Glasgow	3075	3075.00
8	Watt, Graham	Univ of Glasgow	3075	3075.00
9	Wyke, Sally	Univ of Glasgow	3075	3075.00
10	O'Brien, Bridget C.	Univ of Calif, San Francisco	2632	219.33
11	Beckman, Thomas J.	Mayo Clin	2534	133.37
12	Harris, Ilene B.	Univ of Illinois	2407	401.17
13	Shanafelt, Tait D.	Mayo Clin	2361	147.56
14	McGaghie, William C.	Loyola Univ Chicago	2149	85.96
15	West, Colin P.	Mayo Clin	2071	115.06

Figure 19 Authors with the most publications and citations related to medical education between 2011 and 2015

14. Authors with the most publications and citations related to medical education between 2016 and 2020 (Figure 20)

Ranking	Author with the most publicatins	Institution	Number of publications
1	Durning, Steven J.	Uniformed Serv Univ of the Hlth Sci	64
2	Park, Yoon Soo	Univ of Illinois	64
3	Ten Cate, Olle	Univ of Med Ctr Utrecht	64
4	Santen, Sally A.	Virginia Commonwealth Univ	50
5	O'Sullivan, Patricia S.	Univ of Calif, San Francisco	44
6	Konge, Lars	Univ of Copenhagen	42
7	van der Vleuten, Cees	Maastricht Univ	42
8	Teunissen, Pim W.	Maastricht Univ	40
9	Cleland, Jennifer	Nanyang Technol Univ	39
10	Tekian, Ara	Univ of Illinois	39
11	van der Vleuten, Cees P. M.	Maastricht Univ	39
12	Schwartz, Alan	Univ of Illinois	37
13	Lingard, Lorelei	Univ of Western Ontario	36
14	Sandhu, Gurjit	Univ of Michigan	36
15	Regehr, Glenn	Univ of British Columbia	33

Ranking	Author with the most citations	Institution	Number of citations	Average number of citations
1	Ten Cate, Olle	Univ of Med Ctr Utrecht	1467	22.92
2	Englander, Robert	Univ of Minnesota	1145	44.04
3	Carraccio, Carol	Amer Board Pediat Inc	967	37.19
4	Durning, Steven J.	Uniformed Serv Univ of the Hlth Sci	925	14.45
5	Frank, Jason R.	Univ of Ottawa	913	36.52
6	Varpio, Lara	Uniformed Serv Univ of the Hlth Sci	873	29.10
7	Bilimoria, Karl Y.	Northwestern Univ	843	33.72
8	Holmboe, Eric S.	Accreditat Council Grad Med Educ	805	32.20
9	Sherbino, Jonathan	McMaster Univ	786	26.20
10	van der Vleuten, Cees P. M.	Maastricht Univ	735	18.85
11	O'Sullivan, Patricia S.	Univ of Calif, San Francisco	668	15.18
12	Yang, Anthony D.	Northwestern Univ	652	40.75
13	Konge, Lars	Univ of Copenhagen	626	14.90
14	Touchie, Claire	Univ of Ottawa	625	39.06
15	Dyrbye, Liselotte N.	Mayo Clin	623	38.94

Figure 20 Authors with the most publications and citations related to medical education between 2016 and 2020

15. Ranking analysis of authors with the most publications and citations related to medical education between 2001 and 2020 (Figure 21)

Author	Publication ranking				Author	Citation ranking			
	2001—2005	2006—2010	2011—2015	2016—2020		2001—2005	2006—2010	2011—2015	2016—2020
Durning, Steven J.	39	3	2	1	Ten Cate, Olle	1649	7	26	1
Park, Yoon Soo	—	—	35	1	Englander, Robert	161	14 441	342	2
Ten Cate, Olle	799	62	35	1	Carraccio, Carol	139	237	2605	3
Santen, Sally A.	799	2872	103	4	Durning, Steven J.	542	51	17	4
O'Sullivan, Patricia S.	150	18	35	5	Frank, Jason R.	3581	4	671	5
Konge, Lars	—	—	43	6	Varpio, Lara	—	1564	1047	6
van der Vleuten, Cees	7	18	3	6	Bilimoria, Karl Y.	—	4386	2320	7
Teunissen, Pim W.	—	118	31	8	Holmboe, Eric S.	78	14	35	8
Cleland, Jennifer	799	41	120	9	Sherbino, Jonathan	—	49	71	9
Tekian, Ara	799	592	54	9	van der Vleuten, Cees P. M.	1	10	2	10
van der Vleuten, Cees P. M.	1	1	1	9	O'Sullivan, Patricia S.	875	134	80	11
Schwartz, Alan	469	285	144	12	Yang, Anthony D.	—	—	18 374	12
Lingard, Lorelei	16	36	13	13	Konge, Lars	—	—	266	13
Sandhu, Gurjit	—	—	4662	13	Touchie, Claire	4812	10 261	3316	14
Regehr, Glenn	2	10	10	15	Dyrbye, Liselotte N.	—	47	18	15

Figure 21　Ranking analysis of authors with the most publications and citations related to medical education between 2001 and 2020

Research hotspots

1. Highest frequent MeSH terms from publications in medical education between 2001 and 2005 (Figure 22)

Ranking	MeSH Term	Frequency	Percentage	Ranking	MeSH Term	Frequency	Percentage
1	Internship and Residency	1853	6.04	21	Physician-Patient Relations	231	0.75
2	Education, Medical, Undergraduate	1315	4.28	22	Computer-Assisted Instruction	208	0.68
3	Clinical Competence	1140	3.71	23	Emergency Medicine	208	0.68
4	Education, Medical	1052	3.43	24	Career Choice	207	0.67
5	Students, Medical	757	2.47	25	Physicians	204	0.66
6	Education, Medical, Graduate	756	2.46	26	Internet	198	0.65
7	Education, Medical, Continuing	648	2.11	27	Psychiatry	194	0.63
8	Teaching	566	1.84	28	Practice Patterns, Physicians'	191	0.62
9	Family Practice	552	1.80	29	Communication	173	0.56
10	Curriculum	540	1.76	30	Physicians, Family	172	0.56
11	Educational Measurement	505	1.65	31	Primary Health Care	155	0.51
12	Attitude of Health Personnel	493	1.61	32	Radiology	150	0.49
13	General Surgery	484	1.58	33	Specialization	150	0.49
14	Pediatrics	313	1.02	34	Professional Competence	138	0.45
15	Faculty, Medical	289	0.94	35	Learning	134	0.44
16	Schools, Medical	281	0.92	36	Academic Medical Centers	128	0.42
17	Problem-Based Learning	277	0.90	37	Obstetrics	127	0.41
18	Internal Medicine	263	0.86	38	Gynecology	126	0.41
19	Clinical Clerkship	250	0.81	39	Health Knowledge, Attitudes, Practice	126	0.41
20	Medical Staff, Hospital	243	0.79	40	Laparoscopy	126	0.41

Figure 22　Highest frequent MeSH terms from publications in medical education between 2001 and 2005

2. Highest frequent MeSH terms from publications in medical education between 2006 and 2010 (Figure 23)

Ranking	MeSH Term	Frequency	Percentage	Ranking	MeSH Term	Frequency	Percentage
1	Internship and Residency	2945	5.82	21	Computer-Assisted Instruction	361	0.71
2	Clinical Competence	1932	3.82	22	Career Choice	355	0.70
3	Education, Medical	1566	3.09	23	Emergency Medicine	320	0.63
4	Education, Medical, Undergraduate	1558	3.08	24	Internet	306	0.60
5	Students, Medical	1480	2.92	25	Physician-Patient Relations	297	0.59
6	Education, Medical, Graduate	1462	2.89	26	Learning	295	0.58
7	Education, Medical, Continuing	1053	2.08	27	Medical Staff, Hospital	286	0.56
8	Teaching	904	1.79	28	Health Knowledge, Attitudes, Practice	284	0.56
9	Curriculum	895	1.77	29	Laparoscopy	281	0.56
10	Educational Measurement	768	1.52	30	Communication	266	0.53
11	General Surgery	757	1.50	31	Clinical Clerkship	259	0.51
12	Attitude of Health Personnel	731	1.44	32	Professional Competence	254	0.50
13	Schools, Medical	548	1.08	33	Practice Patterns, Physicians'	231	0.46
14	Faculty, Medical	497	0.98	34	Academic Medical Centers	213	0.42
15	Pediatrics	462	0.91	35	Computer Simulation	211	0.42
16	Family Practice	425	0.84	36	Physicians, Family	210	0.41
17	Physicians	422	0.83	37	Anesthesiology	209	0.41
18	Internal Medicine	409	0.81	38	Anatomy	207	0.41
19	Psychiatry	392	0.77	39	Patient Simulation	202	0.40
20	Problem-Based Learning	362	0.72	40	Biomedical Research	197	0.39

Figure 23　Highest frequent MeSH terms from publications in medical education between 2006 and 2010

3. Highest frequent MeSH terms from publications in medical education between 2011 and 2015 (Figure 24)

Ranking	MeSH Term	Frequency	Percentage	Ranking	MeSH Term	Frequency	Percentage
1	Internship and Residency	3947	5.91	21	Emergency Medicine	403	0.60
2	Clinical Competence	2827	4.24	22	Health Knowledge, Attitudes, Practice	397	0.59
3	Students, Medical	2237	3.35	23	Psychiatry	393	0.59
4	Education, Medical	1960	2.94	24	Computer-Assisted Instruction	389	0.58
5	Education, Medical, Undergraduate	1943	2.91	25	Laparoscopy	387	0.58
6	Education, Medical, Graduate	1845	2.76	26	Internal Medicine	367	0.55
7	Education, Medical, Continuing	1205	1.81	27	Clinical Clerkship	362	0.54
8	Curriculum	1161	1.74	28	Problem-Based Learning	356	0.53
9	Educational Measurement	1070	1.60	29	Physician-Patient Relations	332	0.50
10	Attitude of Health Personnel	976	1.46	30	Anatomy	319	0.48
11	Teaching	883	1.32	31	Communication	319	0.48
12	General Surgery	877	1.31	32	Internet	315	0.47
13	Physicians	696	1.04	33	Radiology	308	0.46
14	Faculty, Medical	606	0.91	34	Practice Patterns, Physicians'	293	0.44
15	Pediatrics	560	0.84	35	Medical Staff, Hospital	279	0.42
16	Schools, Medical	554	0.83	36	Biomedical Research	277	0.42
17	Career Choice	474	0.71	37	Professional Competence	271	0.41
18	Learning	452	0.68	38	Anesthesiology	252	0.38
19	Computer Simulation	430	0.64	39	Fellowships and Scholarships	245	0.37
20	Family Practice	417	0.62	40	Quality Improvement	237	0.36

Figure 24　Highest frequent MeSH terms from publications in medical education between 2011 and 2015

4. Highest frequent MeSH terms from publications in medical education between 2016 and 2020 (Figure 25)

Ranking	MeSH Term	Frequency	Percentage	Ranking	MeSH Term	Frequency	Percentage
1	Internship and Residency	5532	7.04	21	Emergency Medicine	447	0.57
2	Clinical Competence	3232	4.11	22	Clinical Clerkship	433	0.55
3	Students, Medical	3193	4.06	23	Fellowships and Scholarships	432	0.55
4	Education, Medical, Graduate	2360	3.00	24	Psychiatry	421	0.54
5	Education, Medical, Undergraduate	2342	2.98	25	Anatomy	420	0.53
				26	Problem-Based Learning	419	0.53
6	Education, Medical	2145	2.73	27	Internal Medicine	413	0.53
7	Curriculum	1578	2.01	28	Health Knowledge, Attitudes, Practice	394	0.50
8	Educational Measurement	1147	1.46				
9	General Surgery	1059	1.35	29	Family Practice	368	0.47
10	Physicians	979	1.25	30	Communication	362	0.46
11	Simulation Training	961	1.22	31	Orthopedics	343	0.44
12	Attitude of Health Personnel	892	1.13	32	Laparoscopy	341	0.43
13	Education, Medical, Continuing	847	1.08	33	Radiology	336	0.43
14	Faculty, Medical	638	0.81	34	Burnout, Professional	332	0.42
15	Pediatrics	593	0.75	35	Quality Improvement	331	0.42
16	Learning	580	0.74	36	Health Personnel	328	0.42
17	Teaching	578	0.74	37	Biomedical Research	326	0.41
18	Schools, Medical	561	0.71	38	Computer-Assisted Instruction	313	0.40
19	Career Choice	558	0.71	39	Competency-Based Education	311	0.40
20	Surgeons	453	0.58	40	Otolaryngology	298	0.38

Figure 25　Highest frequent MeSH terms from publications in medical education between 2016 and 2020

5. Ranking analysis of highest frequent MeSH terms from publications in medical education between 2001 and 2020 (Figure 26)

MeSH Term	Frequency ranking				MeSH Term	Frequency ranking			
	2001—2005	2006—2010	2011—2015	2016—2020		2001—2005	2006—2010	2011—2015	2016—2020
Internship and Residency	1	1	1	1	Emergency Medicine	23	23	21	21
Clinical Competence	3	2	2	2	Clinical Clerkship	19	31	27	22
Students, Medical	5	2	3	3	Fellowships and Scholarships	56	43	39	23
Education, Medical, Graduate	6	3	6	4	Psychiatry	27	19	23	24
Education, Medical, Undergraduate	2	4	5	5	Anatomy	50	38	30	25
Education, Medical	4	3	4	6	Problem-Based Learning	17	20	28	26
Curriculum	10	9	8	7	Internal Medicine	18	18	26	27
Educational Measurement	11	10	9	8	Health Knowledge, Attitudes, Practice	39	28	22	28
General Surgery	13	11	12	9	Family Practice	9	16	20	29
Physicians	25	17	13	10	Communication	29	30	31	30
Simulation Training	—	—	87	11	Orthopedics	68	46	48	31
Attitude of Health Personnel	12	12	10	12	Laparoscopy	40	29	25	32
Education, Medical, Continuing	7	7	7	13	Radiology	32	44	33	33
Faculty, Medical	15	14	14	14	Burnout, Professional	185	148	118	34
Pediatrics	14	15	15	15	Quality Improvement	—	561	40	35
Learning	35	26	18	16	Health Personnel	102	71	43	36
Teaching	8	8	11	17	Biomedical Research	58	40	36	37
Schools, Medical	16	13	16	18	Computer-Assisted Instruction	22	21	24	38
Career Choice	24	22	17	19	Competency-Based Education	59	41	51	39
Surgeons	—	—	166	20	Otolaryngology	112	83	49	40

Figure 26　Ranking analysis of highest frequent MeSH terms from publications in medical education between 2001 and 2020

6. Highest frequent MeSH terms clustering of publications in medical education between 2001 and 2005 (Figure 27)

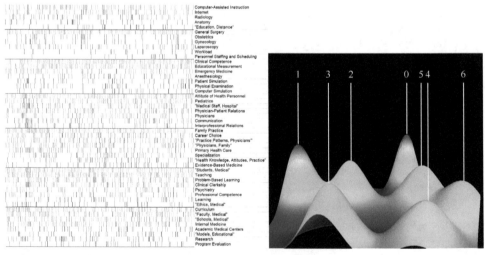

Figure 27　Highest frequent MeSH terms clustering of publications in medical education between 2001 and 2005

Note: The numbers in the right figure indicate the theme categories formed by the highest frequent MeSH terms clustering of publications.

Through highest frequent MeSH terms clustering, six major themes about medical education between 2001 and 2005 have emerged:

(1) Research on Internet-based teaching model and evaluation of medical curricula.

(2) Research on resident workload and its relationship with job satisfaction and health care quality.

(3) The application of simulation-based medical education in clinical skills evaluation and assessment.

(4) Evidence-based medicine and its application in clinical practice.

(5) Research on professionalism among physicians, residents, and medical students.

(6) Others, including evaluation of residency programs and interdisciplinary programs.

7. Highest frequent MeSH terms clustering of publications in medical education between 2006 and 2010 (Figure 28)

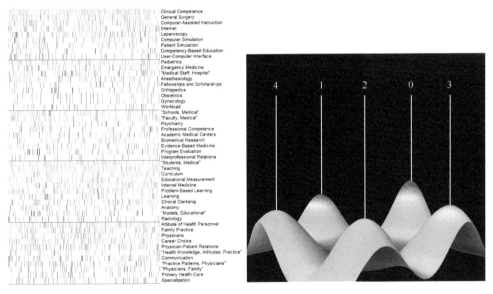

Figure 28   Highest frequent MeSH terms clustering of publications in medical education between 2006 and 2010

Note: The numbers in the right figure indicate the theme categories formed by the highest frequent MeSH terms clustering of publications.

Through highest frequent MeSH terms clustering, five major themes about medical education between 2006 and 2010 have emerged:

(1) The application and evaluation of simulation-based medical education in clinical skills training.

(2) Research on reforms of standardized training systems for residents, especially the rationalization of workloads and the improvement of salary and benefits.

(3) Research on training and improvement of non-technical skills in clinicians and medical students.

(4) Research on the reform of theories, models, and methods for teaching and evaluation.

(5) Others, including choice of specialization for physicians and medical students and the quality improvement of primary care.

8. Highest frequent MeSH terms clustering of publications in medical education between 2011 and 2015 (Figure 29)

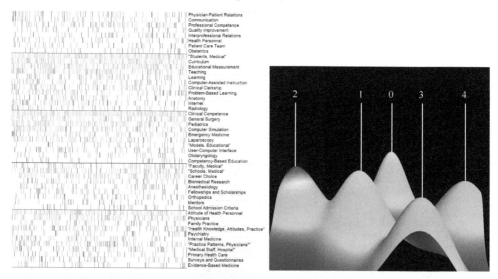

Figure 29　Highest frequent MeSH terms clustering of publications in medical education between 2011 and 2015

Note: The numbers in the right figure indicate the theme categories formed by the highest frequent MeSH terms clustering of publications.

Through highest frequent MeSH terms clustering, five major themes about medical education between 2011 and 2015 have emerged:

(1) Research on the development of clinical interpersonal communication and teamwork skills.

(2) Research on Internet-based teaching and evaluation of medical curricula.

(3) The application of simulation-based medical education in clinical skills training.

(4) Research on academic career development and influencing factors for medical faculty and medical students.

(5) Evidence-based medicine and its application in clinical practice.

9. Highest frequent MeSH terms clustering of publications in medical education between 2016 and 2020 (Figure 30)

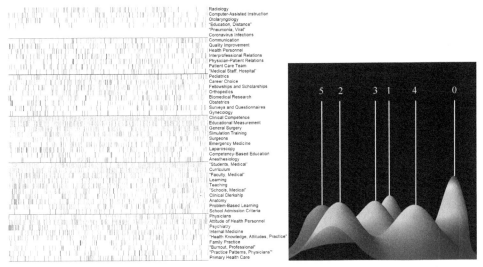

Figure 30　Highest frequent MeSH terms clustering of publications in medical education between
2016 and 2020

Note: The numbers in the right figure indicate the theme categories formed by the highest frequent
MeSH terms clustering of publications.

Through highest frequent MeSH terms clustering, six major themes about medical education between 2016 and 2020 have emerged:

(1) Research on the reform of medical teaching model and method under the influence of the COVID-19 pandemic.

(2) Research on communication in interprofessional healthcare teams.

(3) Research on applications of simulation-based medical education in clinical skills training and evaluation.

(4) Research on student-centered teaching.

(5) Research on physician burnout, influencing factors, and intervention for addressing burnout.

(6) Others, including career choice and performance-based pay distribution.

Ⅲ. Special topic: global research on teaching in medical education

Methods

1. Search Strategy

Search Strategy: "Education, Medical" [MeSH] OR (*Academic Medicine /*

Medical Education / Medical Teacher / BMC Medical Education / Journal of Surgical Education / Advances in Health Sciences Education / Teaching and Learning in Medicine / Medical Education Online / Anatomical Sciences Education / Academic Psychiatry) [Journal] AND "Teaching" [MeSH].

2. Time range

2012-01-01—2021-12-31.

3. Statistical method

CiteSpace was used to analyze bibliometric data, such as the number of publications per country/region, per institution, and per author. High frequency MeSH terms clustering was conducted on the main MeSH terms included in literature from the last decade (2012—2021). Co-citation clustering was performed on the most cited papers from the last decade (2011—2020).

Scope of literature and research fronts

1. Countries/regions with the most publications of research on teaching in medical education in the recent ten years (2012—2021) (Figure 31)

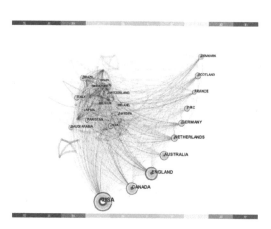

Ranking	Country/Region	Number of publications	Percentage
1	USA	3549	35.51
2	UK	900	9.01
3	Canada	814	8.15
4	Australia	532	5.32
5	Netherlands	381	3.81
6	Germany	326	3.26
7	PRC	209	2.09
8	France	180	1.80
9	Denmark	140	1.40
10	India	122	1.22
11	Brazil	118	1.18
12	Italy	117	1.17
13	Switzerland	116	1.16
14	Japan	110	1.10
15	Saudi Arabia	106	1.06

Figure 31　Countries/regions with the most publications of research on teaching in medical education in the recent ten years (2012—2021)

Note: CiteSpace nodes (left) represent countries/regions (publications per time slice, with size of node reflecting cumulative number of publications). Each ring represents a single time slice (1 year), from blue (2012) to red (2021). Thickness of time slice ring is proportional to the number of publications in that particular time slice (1 year). Links between different countries/regions represent cooperative relationships.

2. Institutions with the most publications of research on teaching in medical education in the recent ten years (2012—2021) (Figure 32)

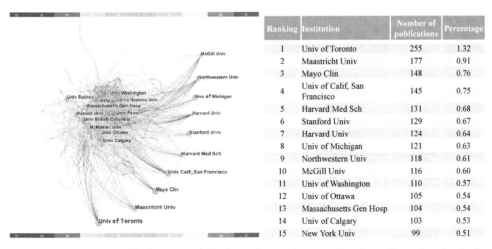

Ranking	Institution	Number of publications	Percentage
1	Univ of Toronto	255	1.32
2	Maastricht Univ	177	0.91
3	Mayo Clin	148	0.76
4	Univ of Calif, San Francisco	145	0.75
5	Harvard Med Sch	131	0.68
6	Stanford Univ	129	0.67
7	Harvard Univ	124	0.64
8	Univ of Michigan	121	0.63
9	Northwestern Univ	118	0.61
10	McGill Univ	116	0.60
11	Univ of Washington	110	0.57
12	Univ of Ottawa	105	0.54
13	Massachusetts Gen Hosp	104	0.54
14	Univ of Calgary	103	0.53
15	New York Univ	99	0.51

Figure 32　Institutions with the most publications of research on teaching in medical education in the recent ten years (2012—2021)

Note: CiteSpace visualization on the left shows the distribution of institutions with the most publications (per time slice of 1 year) and close cooperation between different institutions.

3. Authors with the most publications of research on teaching in medical education in the recent ten years (2012—2021) (Figure 33)

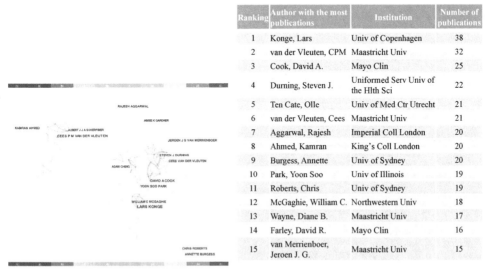

Ranking	Author with the most publications	Institution	Number of publications
1	Konge, Lars	Univ of Copenhagen	38
2	van der Vleuten, CPM	Maastricht Univ	32
3	Cook, David A.	Mayo Clin	25
4	Durning, Steven J.	Uniformed Serv Univ of the Hlth Sci	22
5	Ten Cate, Olle	Univ of Med Ctr Utrecht	21
6	van der Vleuten, Cees	Maastricht Univ	21
7	Aggarwal, Rajesh	Imperial Coll London	20
8	Ahmed, Kamran	King's Coll London	20
9	Burgess, Annette	Univ of Sydney	20
10	Park, Yoon Soo	Univ of Illinois	19
11	Roberts, Chris	Univ of Sydney	19
12	McGaghie, William C.	Northwestern Univ	18
13	Wayne, Diane B.	Maastricht Univ	17
14	Farley, David R.	Mayo Clin	16
15	van Merrienboer, Jeroen J. G.	Maastricht Univ	15

Figure 33　Authors with the most publications of research on teaching in medical education in the recent ten years (2012—2021)

Note: CiteSpace visualization on the left shows the distribution of authors with the most publications (per time slice of 1 year) and close cooperation between different authors.

4. Highest frequent MeSH terms from publications of research on teaching in medical education in the recent ten years (2012—2021) (Figure 34)

Ranking	MeSH Term	Frequency	Percentage	Ranking	MeSH Term	Frequency	Percentage
1	Teaching	2308	5.35	21	Pediatrics	297	0.69
2	Education, Medical, Undergraduate	2196	5.09	22	Communication	271	0.63
3	Education, Medical	1958	4.54	23	Education, Distance	263	0.61
4	Internship and Residency	1929	4.47	24	Attitude of Health Personnel	234	0.54
5	Students, Medical	1884	4.37	25	Internet	233	0.54
6	Clinical Competence	1804	4.18	26	Laparoscopy	232	0.54
7	Simulation Training	1563	3.62	27	Schools, Medical	223	0.52
8	Education, Medical, Graduate	1220	2.83	28	Emergency Medicine	220	0.51
9	Problem-Based Learning	1120	2.60	29	Clinical Clerkship	217	0.50
10	Computer-Assisted Instruction	977	2.26	30	Peer Group	196	0.45
11	Curriculum	963	2.23	31	Radiology	185	0.43
12	Learning	601	1.39	32	Anesthesiology	184	0.43
13	Educational Measurement	555	1.29	33	COVID-19	183	0.42
14	Models, Educational	533	1.24	34	Physicians	182	0.42
15	Patient Simulation	490	1.14	35	Internal Medicine	181	0.42
16	Faculty, Medical	475	1.10	36	Physician-Patient Relations	179	0.41
17	General Surgery	459	1.06	37	Interprofessional Relations	156	0.36
18	Education, Medical, Continuing	435	1.01	38	Competency-Based Education	152	0.35
19	Anatomy	407	0.94	39	Patient Care Team	145	0.34
20	Computer Simulation	302	0.70	40	Psychiatry	143	0.33

Figure 34　Highest frequent MeSH terms from publications of research on teaching in medical education in the recent ten years (2012—2021)

5. Highly cited papers of research on teaching(top1%) in medical education in the recent ten years (2012—2021) (Figure 35)

Ranking	Highly cited papers	Frequency
1	McLaughlin JE, Roth MT, Glatt DM, et al. The flipped classroom: a course redesign to foster learning and engagement in a health professions school. Acad Med, 2014, 89(2):236-243.	541
2	Motola I, Devine LA, Chung HS, et al. Simulation in healthcare education: a best evidence practical guide. AMEE Guide No. 82. Med Teach, 2013, 35(10):e1511-1530.	381
3	Taylor DC, Hamdy H. Adult learning theories: implications for learning and teaching in medical education: AMEE Guide No. 83. Med Teach, 2013, 35(11):e1561-1572.	347
4	Cook DA, Hamstra SJ, Brydges R, et al. Comparative effectiveness of instructional design features in simulation-based education: systematic review and meta-analysis. Med Teach, 2013, 35(1):e867-898.	307
5	Eppich W, Cheng A. Promoting Excellence and Reflective Learning in Simulation (PEARLS): development and rationale for a blended approach to health care simulation debriefing. Simul Healthc, 2015, 10(2):106-115.	286
6	Young JQ, Van Merrienboer J, Durning S, et al. Cognitive Load Theory: implications for medical education: AMEE Guide No. 86. Med Teach, 2014, 36(5):371-384.	282
7	Norman G, Dore K, Grierson L. The minimal relationship between simulation fidelity and transfer of learning. Med Educ, 2012, 46(7):636-647.	281
8	McGaghie WC, Issenberg SB, Barsuk JH, et al. A critical review of simulation-based mastery learning with translational outcomes. Med Educ, 2014, 48(4):375-385.	275
9	Chen F, Lui AM, Martinelli SM. A systematic review of the effectiveness of flipped classrooms in medical education. Med Educ, 2017, 51(6):585-597.	245
10	Hew KF, Lo CK. Flipped classroom improves student learning in health professions education: a meta-analysis. BMC Med Educ, 2018, 18(1):38.	244
11	Ericsson KA. Acquisition and maintenance of medical expertise: a perspective from the expert-performance approach with deliberate practice. Acad Med, 2015, 90(11):1471-1486.	232
12	Moro C, Štromberga Z, Raikos A, et al. The effectiveness of virtual and augmented reality in health sciences and medical anatomy. Anat Sci Educ, 2017, 10(6):549-559.	222
13	Preece D, Williams SB, Lam R, et al. "Let's get physical": advantages of a physical model over 3D computer models and textbooks in learning imaging anatomy. Anat Sci Educ, 2013, 6(4):216-224.	209
14	va KW, Armson H, Holmboe E, et al. Factors influencing responsiveness to feedback: on the interplay between fear, confidence, and reasoning processes. Adv Health Sci Educ Theory Pract, 2012, 17(1):15-26.	209
15	Dedeilia A, Sotiropoulos MG, Hanrahan JG, et al. Medical and surgical education challenges and innovations in the COVID-19 era: a systematic review. In Vivo, 2020, 34(3 Suppl):1603-1611.	173
16	Osseo-Asare A, Balasuriya L, Huot SJ, et al. Minority resident physicians' views on the role of race/Ethnicity in their training experiences in the workplace. JAMA Network Open, 2018, 1(5):e182723.	160
17	Yammine K, Violato C. A meta-analysis of the educational effectiveness of three-dimensional visualization technologies in teaching anatomy. Anat Sci Educ, 2015, 8(6):525-538.	128
18	Pather N, Blyth P, Chapman JA, et al. Forced disruption of anatomy education in Australia and New Zealand: an acute response to the COVID-19 pandemic. Anat Sci Educ, 2020, 13(3):284-300.	125
19	Pei L, Wu H. Does online learning work better than offline learning in undergraduate medical education? A systematic review and meta-analysis. Med Educ Online, 2019, 24(1):1666538.	122
20	Trelease RB. From chalkboard, slides, and paper to e-learning: how computing technologies have transformed anatomical sciences education. Anat Sci Educ, 2016, 9(6):583-602.	109
21	Al-Balas M, Al-Balas HI, Jaber HM, et al. Distance learning in clinical medical education amid COVID-19 pandemic in Jordan: current situation, challenges, and perspectives. BMC Med Educ, 2020, 20(1):341.	104
22	Kogan M, Klein SE, Hannon CP, et al. Orthopaedic education during the COVID-19 pandemic. J Am Acad Orthop Surg, 2020, 28(11):456-464.	101
23	Gorbanev I, Agudelo-Londoño S, González RA, et al. A systematic review of serious games in medical education: quality of evidence and pedagogical strategy. Med Educ Online, 2018, 23(1):1438718.	74
24	Zhao J, Xu X, Jiang H, et al. The effectiveness of virtual reality-based technology on anatomy teaching: a meta-analysis of randomized controlled studies. BMC Med Educ, 2020, 20(1):127.	38
25	Harmon DJ, Attardi SM, Barremkala M, et al. An analysis of anatomy education before and during COVID-19: May-August 2020. Anat Sci Educ, 2021, 14(2):132-147.	27
26	Jiang Z, Wu H, Cheng H, et al. Twelve tips for teaching medical students online under COVID-19. Med Educ Online, 2021, 26(1):1854066.	22
27	Jack MM, Gattozzi DA, Camarata PJ, et al. Live-streaming surgery for medical student education - educational solutions in neurosurgery during the COVID-19 Pandemic. J Surg Educ, 2021, 78(1):99-103.	16

Figure 35　Highly cited papers of research on teaching(top1%) in medical education in the recent ten years (2012—2021)

6. Highest frequent MeSH terms clustering of publications of research on teaching in medical education in the recent three years (2012—2021) (Figure 36)

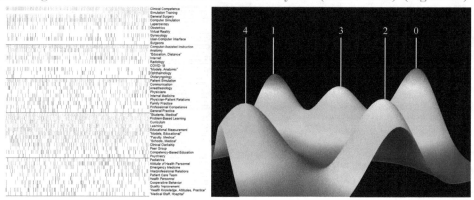

Figure 36   Highest frequent MeSH terms clustering of publications of research on teaching in medical education in the recent three years (2012—2021)

Note: The numbers in the right figure indicate the theme categories formed by the highest frequent MeSH terms clustering of publications.

Through highest frequent MeSH terms clustering, five major themes of research on teaching in medical education emerged:

(1) The application of simulation-based medical education in clinical skills training.

(2) Research on the reform of medical teaching models and methods under the influence of the COVID-19 pandemic.

(3) Research on strategies and methods for physician-patient communication skills training.

(4) Research on competency-oriented teaching and evaluation.

(5) Research on interprofessional education and development of teamwork skills.

7. Co-citation clustering of research on teaching in medical education in the recent ten years (2011—2020) (Figure 37)

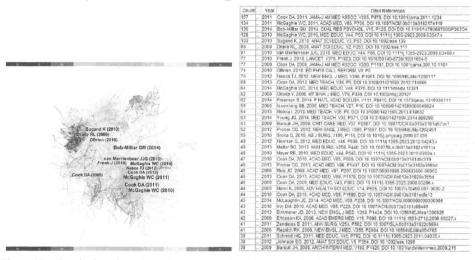

Figure 37   Co-citation clustering of research on teaching in medical education in the recent ten years (2011—2020)

Based on co-citation clustering, highly cited papers in medical educational technology in the recent ten years were classified into the following seven major themes:

(1) Simulation-based medical education, especially research and applications of virtual patients.

Recommended reading:

[1] McGaghie W C, Issenberg S B, Barsuk J H, et al. A critical review of simulation-based mastery learning with translational outcomes. Med Educ, 2014, 48(4): 375-385.

[2] Cook D A, Hamstra S J, Brydges R, et al. Comparative effectiveness of instructional design features in simulation-based education: systematic review and meta-analysis. Med Teach, 2013, 35(1): e867-898.

[3] Cook D A, Hatala R, Brydges R, et al. Technology-enhanced simulation for health professions education: a systematic review and meta-analysis. JAMA, 2011, 306(9): 978-988.

[4] McGaghie W C, Issenberg S B, Cohen E R, et al. Does simulation-based medical education with deliberate practice yield better results than traditional clinical education? A meta-analytic comparative review of the evidence. Acad Med, 2011, 86(6): 706-711.

[5] McGaghie W C, Issenberg S B, Petrusa E R, et al. A critical review of simulation-based medical education research: 2003-2009. Med Educ, 2010, 44(1): 50-63.

[6] Okuda Y, Bryson E O, DeMaria S Jr, et al. The utility of simulation in medical education: what is the evidence?. Mt Sinai J Med, 2009, 76(4), 330-343.

[7] Cook D A, Erwin P J, Triola M M. Computerized virtual patients in health professions education: a systematic review and meta-analysis. Acad Med, 2010, 85(10): 1589-1602.

[8] Cook D A, Triola M M. Virtual patients: a critical literature review and proposed next steps. Med Educ, 2009, 43(4): 303-311.

(2) Research on teaching methods emphasizing self-directed learning.

Recommended reading:

[1] Freeman S, Eddy S L, McDonough M, et al. Active learning increases student performance in science, engineering, and mathematics. Proc Natl Acad Sci U S A, 2014, 111(23): 8410-8415.

[2] McLaughlin J E, Roth M T, Glatt D M, et al. The flipped classroom: a course redesign to foster learning and engagement in a health professions school. Acad Med, 2014, 89(2): 236-243.

[3] Mann K, Gordon J, MacLeod A. Reflection and reflective practice in health professions education: a systematic review. Adv Health Sci Educ Theory Pract, 2009, 14(4): 595-621.

(3) Research, practice, and implications of theories related to medical education.

Recommended reading:

[1] Young J Q, Van Merrienboer J, Durning S, et al. Cognitive load theory: implications for medical education: AMEE Guide No. 86. Med Teach, 2014, 36(5): 371-384.

[2] van Merriënboer J J, Sweller J. Cognitive load theory in health professional education: design principles and strategies. Med Educ, 2010, 44(1): 85-93.

[3] Mayer R E. Applying the science of learning to medical education. Med Educ, 2010, 44(6): 543-549.

(4) The application of Internet-based learning in medical education.

Recommended reading:

[1] Cook D A, Levinson A J, Garside S, et al. Internet-based learning in the health professions: a meta-analysis. JAMA, 2008, 300(10): 1181-1196.

[2] Cook D A, Levinson A J, Garside S, et al. Instructional design variations in Internet-based learning for health professions education: a systematic review and meta-analysis. Acad Med, 2010, 85(5): 909-922.

[3] Ruiz J G, Mintzer M J, Leipzig R M. The impact of E-learning in medical education. Acad Med, 2006, 81(3): 207-212.

(5) Research on the reform of medical education teaching and evaluation.

Recommended reading:

[1] Prober C G, Khan S. Medical education reimagined: a call to action. Acad Med, 2013, 88(10): 1407-1410.

[2] Nasca T J, Philibert I, Brigham T, et al. The next GME accreditation system—rationale and benefits. N Engl J Med, 2012, 366(11): 1051-1056.

[3] Irby D M, Cooke M, O'Brien B C. Calls for reform of medical education by the Carnegie Foundation for the Advancement of Teaching: 1910 and 2010. Acad Med, 2010, 85(2): 220-227.

[4] Frenk J, Chen L, Bhutta Z A, et al. Health professionals for a new century: transforming education to strengthen health systems in an interdependent world. Lancet, 2010, 376(9756): 1923-1958.

(6) Research on surgical skills training and its relationship with health care quality.

Recommended reading:

[1] Julià D, Gómez N, Codina-Cazador A. Surgical skill and complication rates after bariatric surgery. N Engl J Med, 2014, 370(3): 285.

[2] Mattar S G, Alseidi A A, Jones D B, et al. General surgery residency inadequately prepares trainees for fellowship: results of a survey of fellowship program directors. Ann Surg, 2013, 258(3): 440-449.

[3] Sroka G, Feldman L S, Vassiliou M C, et al. Fundamentals of laparoscopic surgery simulator training to proficiency improves laparoscopic performance in the operating room—a randomized controlled trial. Am J Surg, 2010, 199(1): 115-120.

[4] Reznick R K, MacRae H. Teaching surgical skills—changes in the wind. N Engl J Med, 2006, 355(25): 2664-2669.

(7) The modernization of anatomy courses, especially the reform of teaching models and methods.

Recommended reading:

[1] Johnson E O, Charchanti A V, Troupis T G. Modernization of an anatomy class: from conceptualization to implementation. A case for integrated multimodal-multidisciplinary teaching. Anat Sci Educ, 2012, 5(6): 354-366.

[2] Sugand K, Abrahams P, Khurana A. The anatomy of anatomy: a review for its modernization. Anat Sci Educ, 2010, 3(2): 83-93.

[3] Drake R L, McBride J M, Lachman N, et al. Medical education in the anatomical sciences: the winds of change continue to blow. Anat Sci Educ, 2009, 2(6): 253-259.

Ⅳ. ESI ranking of medical education

ESI (Essential Science Indicators) is a basic analysis and assessment tool launched by Thomson Reuters Corporation, a world-famous academic information database corporation, to measure scientific research performance and track scientific development trends. It is a scientometrics database of more than 12 million articles from more than 12,000 academic journals in the world, collected by Web of Science and including the Science Citation Index (SCI) and Social Science Citation Index (SSCI) databases. From the perspective of citation analysis, ESI categorizes 22 professional disciplines for statistical analysis and ranks by country/region, institution, journal, paper, and author. ESI has become one of the most important evaluation indices used to assess the academic level and influence of universities, academic institutions, and countries/regions around the world.

The total number of citations of an institution is an important indicator of the institution's research ability and influence. One of China's major strategic decisions was to build world-class universities and specializations, which would enhance the overall strength and global competitiveness of China's higher education sector. In this regard, ESI rankings would be an important indicator of world-class universities and specialties. Therefore, we have introduced the concept of ESI ranking into the field of medical education research through cooperation with Clarivate and established ESI statistical analysis and ranking of research institutions for medical education. By introducing the ESI ranking of medical education research institutions, we can encourage higher-ranked institutions to improve on existing strengths and also find gaps among different institutions, thereby paving the way for future research and practice.

In the 2019 International Medical Education Research Fronts Report, we issued the ESI institution ranking of medical education for the first time, which has been widely praised and welcomed. In 2022, we continue to update the ESI institution ranking of medical education and compare with the ESI ranking issued in the previous two years to provide better reference data for global scholars.

Methods

1. Search Strategy

"Education, Medical" [MeSH] AND (*Academic Medicine / Medical Education / Medical Teacher / BMC Medical Education / Journal of Surgical Education / Advances in Health Sciences Education / Teaching and Learning in Medicine / Medical Education Online / Anatomical Sciences Education / Academic Psychiatry*) [Journal].

2. Time Range

2012-01-01—2021-12-31.

3. Statistical Method

The total citation count of publications included in the retrieval scope was calculated for each institution. Total citation count reflected academic impact.

Ranking of medical education research institutions by ESI

1. Top 1‰ medical education research institutions by ESI(23/23286) (Figure 38)

Ranking	ESI institution	Country	Number of citations	Number of publications	Average number of citations	ESI ranking in 2020	ESI ranking in 2021	ESI ranking in 2022
1	Univ of Toronto	Canada	12 845	1535	8.37	1	1	1
2	Mayo Clin	USA	9776	1025	9.54	3	2	2
3	Harvard Univ	USA	9260	799	11.59	2	3	3
4	Univ of Calif, San Francisco	USA	8885	1259	7.06	4	4	4
5	Univ of Michigan	USA	6993	1112	6.29	7	6	5
6	Univ of Penn	USA	6691	961	6.96	9	9	6
7	Maastricht Univ	Netherlands	6408	736	8.71	5	5	7
8	Univ of Washington	USA	6354	879	7.23	13	11	8
9	Univ of British Columbia	Canada	6253	686	9.12	8	7	9
10	Stanford Univ	USA	6079	895	6.79	12	12	10
11	Univ of Ottawa	Canada	6027	625	9.64	10	10	11
12	Northwestern Univ	USA	5782	748	7.73	6	8	12
13	Johns Hopkins Univ	USA	5217	769	6.78	14	13	13
14	Massachusetts Gen Hosp	USA	5041	707	7.13	17	16	14
15	McGill Univ	Canada	4810	556	8.65	15	15	15
16	McMaster Univ	Canada	4562	574	7.95	11	17	16
17	Yale Univ	USA	4561	550	8.29	16	14	17
18	Vanderbilt Univ	USA	4464	644	6.93	19	20	18
19	Duke Univ	USA	4409	619	7.12	18	18	19
20	Brigham & Women's Hosp	USA	4241	603	7.03	20	19	20
21	Oregon Hlth & Sci Univ	USA	4002	561	7.13	23	22	21
22	Univ of Calgary	Canada	3898	517	7.54	22	21	22
23	Univ of Pittsburgh	USA	3711	560	6.63	21	23	23

Figure 38　Top 1‰ medical education research institutions by ESI

2. Top 10 medical education research institutions in North America by ESI ranking (Figure 39)

Ranking	Global top 1%	Institution	Country	Number of citations	Number of publications	Average number of citations	ESI ranking in 2020	ESI ranking in2021	ESI ranking in 2022
1	√	Univ of Toronto	Canada	12 845	1535	8.37	1	1	1
2	√	Mayo Clin	USA	9776	1025	9.54	3	2	2
3	√	Harvard Univ	USA	9260	799	11.59	2	3	3
4	√	Univ of Calif, San Francisco	USA	8885	1259	7.06	4	4	4
5	√	Univ of Michigan	USA	6993	1112	6.29	7	6	5
6	√	Univ of Penn	USA	6691	961	6.96	9	9	6
7	√	Univ of Washington	USA	6354	879	7.23	13	11	8
8	√	Univ of British Columbia	Canada	6253	686	9.12	8	7	9
9	√	Stanford Univ	USA	6079	895	6.79	12	12	10
10	√	Univ of Ottawa	Canada	6027	625	9.64	10	10	11

Figure 39　Top 10 medical education research institutions in North America by ESI ranking

3. Top 10 medical education research institutions in Europe by ESI ranking (Figure 40)

Ranking	Global top 1%	Institution	Country	Number of citations	Number of publications	Average number of citations	ESI ranking in 2020	ESI ranking in 2021	ESI ranking in 2022
1	√	Maastricht Univ	Netherlands	6408	736	8.71	5	5	7
2	√	Univ of Dundee	UK	3294	197	16.72	29	31	29
3	√	Imperial Coll London	UK	2386	215	11.10	28	40	48
4	√	Univ of Glasgow	UK	2363	105	22.50	58	54	49
5	√	Univ of Med Ctr Utrecht	Netherlands	2101	213	9.86	54	55	53
6	√	Univ College London	UK	1938	328	5.91	64	65	61
7	√	King's Coll London	UK	1862	342	5.44	67	64	67
8	√	Univ of Amsterdam	Netherlands	1853	200	9.27	57	61	70
9	√	Radboud Univ Nijmegen	Netherlands	1459	208	7.01	88	84	84
10	√	Univ of Oxford	UK	1334	275	4.85	97	87	91

Figure 40　Top 10 medical education research institutions in Europe by ESI ranking

4. Top 10 medical education research institutions in Oceania by ESI ranking (Figure 41)

Ranking	Global top 1%	Institution	Country	Number of citations	Number of publications	Average number of citations	ESI ranking in 2020	ESI ranking in 2021	ESI ranking in 2022
1	√	Univ of Melbourne	Australia	2807	337	8.33	42	39	39
2	√	Univ of Sydney	Australia	2754	373	7.38	44	41	40
3	√	Monash Univ	Australia	2658	401	6.63	48	43	44
4	√	Flinders Univ	Australia	1709	199	8.59	79	73	75
5	√	Univ of Queensland	Australia	1626	242	6.72	69	75	78
6	√	Univ of Otago	New Zealand	911	165	5.52	190	153	139
7	√	Univ of Western Australia	Australia	883	142	6.22	177	139	144
8	√	Univ of Auckland	New Zealand	856	161	5.32	141	129	147
9	√	Univ of Adelaide	Australia	771	127	6.07	203	163	159
10	√	Griffith Univ	Australia	717	110	6.52	247	195	171

Figure 41　Top 10 medical education research institutions in Oceania by ESI ranking

5. Top 10 medical education research institutions in Asia by ESI ranking (Figure 42)

Ranking	Global top 1%	Institution	Country	Number of citations	Number of publications	Average number of citations	ESI ranking in 2020	ESI ranking in 2021	ESI ranking in 2022
1	√	King Saud Univ	Saudi Arabia	977	151	6.47	165	132	124
2	√	Natl Univ of Singapore	Singapore	778	174	4.47	265	162	157
3	√	Univ of Hong Kong	PRC	566	91	6.22	239	220	209
4		Yonsei Univ	Republic of Korea	419	44	9.52	298	258	269
5		King Abdulaziz Univ	Saudi Arabia	330	85	3.88	449	381	326
6		King Saud Bin Abdulaziz Univ Hlth Sci	Saudi Arabia	326	57	5.72	389	339	327
7		Natl Univ of Singapore Hosp	Singapore	321	72	4.46	427	334	332
8		All India Inst Med Sci	India	315	108	2.92	652	433	344
9		Chinese Univ of Hong Kong	PRC	297	45	6.60	321	428	368
10		Taiwan Univ	PRC	284	60	4.73	395	375	383

Figure 42　Top 10 medical education research institutions in Asia by ESI ranking

6. Top 10 medical education research institutions in Africa by ESI ranking (Figure 43)

Ranking	Global top 1%	Institution	Country	Number of citations	Number of publications	Average number of citations	ESI ranking in 2020	ESI ranking in 2021	ESI ranking in 2022
1	√	Univ of Cape Town	South Africa	578	103	5.61	153	125	206
2		Stellenbosch Univ	South Africa	499	51	9.78	227	218	238
3		Makerere Univ	Uganda	349	56	6.23	212	211	313
4		Univ of Kwazulu Natal	South Africa	298	69	4.32	413	393	366
5		Univ of Ghana	Ghana	276	19	14.53	467	416	394
6		Univ of Malawi	Malawi	217	33	6.58	378	329	494
7		Univ of Western Cape	South Africa	194	21	9.24	723	598	538
8		Univ of Witwatersrand	South Africa	157	54	2.91	761	696	660
9		Muhimbili Univ of Hlth & Allied Sci	Tanzania	149	26	5.73	933	800	684
10		Univ of Nairobi	Kenya	149	27	5.52	963	811	684

Figure 43　Top 10 medical education research institutions in Africa by ESI ranking

7. Top 10 medical education research institutions in South America by ESI ranking (Figure 44)

Ranking	Global top 1%	Institution	Country	Number of citations	Number of publications	Average number of citations	ESI ranking in 2020	ESI ranking in 2021	ESI ranking in 2022
1	√	Univ of Sao Paulo	Brazil	609	145	4.20	222	213	202
2		Pontificia Catholic Univ of Chile	Chile	335	98	3.42	312	357	323
3		Fed Univ of Sao Paulo	Brazil	269	46	5.85	330	430	404
4		Hosp Clin Porto Alegre	Brazil	268	6	44.67	510	458	407
5		Univ of Peruana Cayetano Heredia	Peru	185	26	7.12	125	596	569
6		Fed Univ of Uberlandia	Brazil	177	13	13.62	561	654	586
7		State Univ of Campinas	Brazil	155	46	3.37	999	766	670
8		Hcor Hosp Coracao	Brazil	89	2	44.50	1320	1211	1049
9		Fed Univ of Minas Gerais	Brazil	75	30	2.50	1574	1284	1197
10		Univ of Chile	Chile	67	35	1.91	1160	1390	1310

Figure 44　Top 10 medical education research institutions in South America by ESI ranking

8. Top 20 medical education research institutions in PRC by ESI ranking (Figure 45)

Ranking	Global top 1%	Institution	Number of citations	Number of publications	Average number of citations	ESI ranking in 2020	ESI ranking in 2021	ESI ranking in 2022
1	√	Univ of Hong Kong	566	91	6.22	239	220	209
2		Chinese Univ of Hong Kong	297	45	6.60	321	428	368
3		Taiwan Univ	284	60	4.73	395	375	383
4		Peking Univ	264	68	3.88	115	452	423
5		Taiwan Univ Hosp	246	49	5.02	523	502	454
6		Sichuan Univ	209	39	5.36	581	450	512
7		Chang Gung Univ	207	74	2.80	736	581	518
8		Chang Gung Mem Hosp	186	48	3.88	816	614	566
9		Yang Ming Univ	167	47	3.55	781	676	623
10		China Med Univ	129	35	3.69	816	867	761
11		Zhejiang Univ	129	20	6.45	1039	902	761
12		Jiangsu Inst of Parasit Dis	121	2	60.50	1023	913	798
13		Army Med Univ	120	41	2.93	1009	883	806
14		Sun Yat-sen Univ	116	40	2.90	993	883	839
15		Capital Med Univ	107	32	3.34	1173	1008	888
16		Air Force Med Univ	97	14	6.93	1589	1315	969
17		Shanghai Jiao Tong Univ	91	34	2.68	1219	1068	1028
18		Fudan Univ	84	41	2.05	1383	1134	1100
19		Cent South Univ	84	22	3.82	1436	1242	1100
20		Taipei Med Univ	76	41	1.85	1838	1390	1181

Figure 45　Top 20 medical education research institutions in PRC by ESI ranking

V. Analysis of medical education journals

Methods

From all journals under the education category (including 44 journals in SCIE and 267 journals in SSCI) of the JCR database, journals on medical education were selected based on the following inclusion criteria.

Inclusion criteria: The journal was considered to be a journal in medical education if 50% or more of its articles published in the recent 10 years (2011-01-01—2020-12-31) were indexed with "Education, Medical" [MeSH].

BICOMB was used to analyze the distribution of high frequent MeSH terms of all journals in medical education in the past ten years (2011-01-01—2020-12-31) to reflect research content and special topics of each journal.

Medical Education Journals (Figure 46)

Ranking	Journal	Database	JCR partition of CAS in 2021* (updated version)	Impact factor (2020)	Country of publication	Number of publications (2011-2020)	Number of papers indexed with "Education, Medical" [MeSH]	Percentage of papers indexed with "Education, Medical" [MeSH]
1	Academic Medicine	SCIE	1	6.893	USA	4870	2515	51.64
2	Medical Education	SCIE	1	6.251	UK	5451	3228	59.22
3	Anatomical Sciences Education	SCIE	1	5.958	USA	703	365	51.92
4	Advances in Health Sciences Education	SCIE/SSCI	1	3.853	USA	775	383	49.42
5	Medical Teacher	SCIE	2	3.650	UK	3166	1907	60.23
6	Medical Education Online	SSCI	3	3.298	UK	596	394	66.11
7	Journal of Surgical Education	SCIE	3	2.891	USA	2078	1592	76.61
8	BMC Medical Education	SCIE/SSCI	3	2.463	UK	2837	1561	55.02
9	Teaching and Learning in Medicine	SCIE	3	2.414	USA	583	386	66.20
10	Academic Psychiatry	SSCI	4	3.293	USA	1645	972	59.09

*SCIE (EDUCATION, SCIENTIFIC DISCIPLINES) /SSCI (EDUCATION & EDUCATIONAL RESEARCH)

Figure 46   Medical education and research journals

Highest frequent MeSH terms per medical education journal

1. *Academic Medicine* (Figure 47)

Ranking	MeSH Term	Frequency	Percentage (A)	A/O①	Ranking	MeSH Term	Frequency	Percentage (A)	A/O①
1	Education, Medical	605	6.99	1.49	16	Curriculum	97	1.12	1.55
2	Students, Medical	516	5.96	1.66	17	Competency-Based Education	86	0.99	2.79
3	Education, Medical, Undergraduate	420	4.85	1.45	18	Teaching	82	0.95	0.73
4	Internship and Residency	358	4.14	0.82	19	Pediatrics	70	0.81	0.43
5	Physicians	296	3.42	2.33	20	Health Personnel	63	0.73	1.38
6	Education, Medical, Graduate	290	3.35	0.84	21	Family Practice	60	0.69	0.92
7	Schools, Medical	264	3.05	3.73	22	Health Occupations	59	0.68	3.34
8	Faculty, Medical	223	2.58	3.51	23	Research Personnel	48	0.55	5.59
9	Educational Measurement	214	2.47	1.46	24	Minority Groups	47	0.54	6.59
10	Academic Medical Centers	188	2.17	8.15	25	Patient Care Team	44	0.51	1.86
11	Internal Medicine	177	2.05	2.37	26	General Surgery	44	0.51	0.25
12	Clinical Competence	140	1.62	0.85	27	Burnout, Professional	44	0.51	1.37
13	Biomedical Research	127	1.47	2.34	28	Physicians, Primary Care	43	0.50	3.13
14	Delivery of Health Care	101	1.17	3.47	29	Problem-Based Learning	41	0.47	0.98
15	Clinical Clerkship	99	1.14	2.51	30	Staff Development	41	0.47	3.17

Figure 47   Highest frequent MeSH terms of *Academic Medicine*

① A/O: A represents the percentage of the occurrence of the corresponding MeSH terms in all papers published in this journal; O represents the percentage of occurrence of the corresponding MeSH terms in all papers indexed with "Education, Medical"[MeSH] in the PubMed database; A/O is the ratio used to measure the publication tendency of the corresponding MeSH terms in this journal. The higher the value, the greater the proportion of the corresponding MeSH terms in this journal, which then provides reference for medical education researchers in selecting the most suitable journal for article submission (Those with A/O >5 have been marked in red, which represent areas of focus).

2. *Medical Education* (Figure 48)

Ranking	MeSH Term	Frequency	Percentage (A)	A/O	Ranking	MeSH Term	Frequency	Percentage (A)	A/O
1	Students, Medical	955	10.20	2.84	16	Health Occupations	76	0.81	4.05
2	Education, Medical, Undergraduate	602	6.43	1.93	17	Computer-Assisted Instruction	74	0.79	1.76
3	Education, Medical	580	6.19	1.32	18	Pediatrics	69	0.74	0.62
4	Clinical Competence	429	4.58	2.40	19	Biomedical Research	67	0.72	1.14
5	Educational Measurement	368	3.93	2.31	20	Medical Staff, Hospital	67	0.72	1.80
					21	General Practice	63	0.67	1.52
6	Internship and Residency	194	2.07	0.41	22	Stress, Psychological	61	0.65	2.71
					23	Curriculum	58	0.62	0.86
7	Teaching	181	1.93	1.50	24	Education, Medical, Continuing	57	0.61	0.37
8	Education, Medical, Graduate	151	1.61	0.40	25	Professional Competence	57	0.61	3.81
9	Problem-Based Learning	148	1.58	3.31	26	Competency-Based Education	53	0.57	1.63
10	Physicians	143	1.53	1.04	27	Evidence-Based Medicine	48	0.51	2.55
11	Health Personnel	116	1.24	2.34					
12	Schools, Medical	115	1.23	1.50	28	Students, Health Occupations	47	0.50	4.55
13	Faculty, Medical	97	1.04	1.42	29	Family Practice	45	0.48	0.64
14	Internal Medicine	96	1.03	1.20	30	Students, Nursing	42	0.45	5.00
15	Clinical Clerkship	82	0.88	1.96					

Figure 48   Highest frequent MeSH terms of *Medical Education*

3. *Anatomical Sciences Education* (Figure 49)

Ranking	MeSH Term	Frequency	Percentage (A)	A/O	Ranking	MeSH Term	Frequency	Percentage (A)	A/O
1	Anatomy	529	26.21	33.18	16	Tissue and Organ Procurement	19	0.94	31.33
2	Education, Medical, Undergraduate	204	10.11	3.03	17	Tissue Donors	18	0.89	29.67
3	Students, Medical	153	7.58	2.11	18	Health Occupations	17	0.84	4.20
4	Teaching	120	5.95	4.61	19	Education, Professional	16	0.79	11.29
5	Dissection	63	3.12	20.80	20	Anatomists	14	0.69	34.50
6	Educational Measurement	46	2.28	1.34	21	Physical Therapy Specialty	12	0.59	9.83
7	Computer-Assisted Instruction	46	2.28	5.07	22	Faculty	11	0.55	5.00
					23	Education, Distance	10	0.50	1.85
8	Education, Medical	38	1.88	0.40	24	Anatomy, Regional	9	0.45	22.50
9	Students	32	1.59	12.23	25	Anatomy, Cross-Sectional	9	0.45	45.00
10	Histology	29	1.44	36.00					
11	Problem-Based Learning	28	1.39	2.90	26	Radiology	9	0.45	0.58
12	Neuroanatomy	25	1.24	31.00	27	Physiology	8	0.40	4.00
13	Curriculum	23	1.14	1.58	28	Education, Veterinary	8	0.40	13.33
14	Students, Health Occupations	21	1.04	9.45	29	Education, Medical, Graduate	8	0.40	0.10
15	Schools, Medical	21	1.04	1.27	30	Imaging, Three-Dimensional	7	0.35	11.67

Figure 49   Highest frequent MeSH terms of *Anatomical Sciences Education*

4. *Advances in Health Sciences Education* (Figure 50)

Ranking	MeSH Term	Frequency	Percentage (A)	A/O	Ranking	MeSH Term	Frequency	Percentage (A)	A/O
1	Students, Medical	124	9.23	2.57	16	Science	15	1.12	7.00
2	Educational Measurement	102	7.59	4.46	17	Students, Health Occupations	15	1.12	10.18
3	Education, Medical	87	6.48	1.38	18	Clinical Clerkship	14	1.04	2.31
4	Education, Medical, Undergraduate	61	4.54	1.36	19	Internal Medicine	13	0.97	1.13
5	Health Occupations	44	3.28	16.40	20	School Admission Criteria	13	0.97	10.78
6	Clinical Competence	40	2.98	1.56	21	Workplace	11	0.82	10.51
7	Schools, Medical	35	2.60	3.17	22	Competency-Based Education	11	0.82	1.82
8	Problem-Based Learning	35	2.60	5.42	23	Computer-Assisted Instruction	10	0.74	1.64
9	Teaching	34	2.53	1.96	24	Cardiology	9	0.67	1.56
10	Physicians	30	2.23	1.52	25	Students, Nursing	8	0.60	6.67
11	Education, Medical, Graduate	26	1.94	0.49	26	Students	8	0.60	4.62
12	Health Personnel	26	1.94	3.66	27	Licensure, Medical	8	0.60	6.67
13	Internship and Residency	24	1.79	0.36	28	Physical Therapy Specialty	8	0.60	10.00
14	Research	18	1.34	9.57	29	Staff Development	8	0.60	4.00
15	Faculty, Medical	18	1.34	1.84	30	Patient Care Team	8	0.60	2.22

Figure 50　Highest frequent MeSH terms of *Advances in Health Sciences Education*

5. *Medical Teacher* (Figure 51)

Ranking	MeSH Term	Frequency	Percentage (A)	A/O	Ranking	MeSH Term	Frequency	Percentage (A)	A/O
1	Education, Medical	520	11.54	2.47	16	Health Occupations	41	0.91	4.55
2	Students, Medical	499	11.07	3.08	17	Staff Development	40	0.89	5.93
3	Education, Medical, Undergraduate	393	8.72	2.61	18	Education, Distance	34	0.75	2.78
4	Educational Measurement	259	5.75	3.38	19	Internal Medicine	33	0.73	0.85
					20	Medical Staff, Hospital	31	0.69	1.64
5	Teaching	194	4.31	3.34	21	Curriculum	30	0.67	0.93
6	Schools, Medical	119	2.64	3.22	22	Computer-Assisted Instruction	29	0.64	1.42
7	Clinical Competence	106	2.35	1.23					
8	Faculty, Medical	99	2.20	3.01	23	Professionalism	25	0.55	3.93
9	Internship and Residency	99	2.20	0.44	24	Pediatrics	24	0.53	0.45
10	Health Personnel	92	2.04	3.85	25	Program Evaluation	24	0.53	4.82
11	Problem-Based Learning	89	1.98	4.13	26	Professional Competence	23	0.51	3.19
12	Education, Medical, Graduate	73	1.62	0.41	27	Research	23	0.51	3.64
13	Clinical Clerkship	71	1.58	3.51	28	Education, Medical, Continuing	22	0.49	0.29
14	Physicians	63	1.40	0.95	29	Education, Professional	21	0.47	6.71
15	Competency-Based Education	48	1.07	3.06	30	Simulation Training	20	0.44	0.56

Figure 51　Highest frequent MeSH terms of *Medical Teacher*

6. *Medical Education Online* (Figure 52)

Ranking	MeSH Term	Frequency	Percentage (A)	A/O	Ranking	MeSH Term	Frequency	Percentage (A)	A/O
1	Students, Medical	140	11.71	3.26	16	Coronavirus Infections	12	1.00	1.67
2	Education, Medical, Undergraduate	95	7.94	2.28	17	Pneumonia, Viral	12	1.00	0.83
3	Education, Medical	80	6.69	1.43	18	Biomedical Research	11	0.92	1.46
4	Internship and Residency	62	5.18	1.03	19	Education, Distance	11	0.92	3.41
					20	Emergency Medicine	10	0.84	0.93
5	Educational Measurement	54	4.52	2.66	21	Health Personnel	9	0.75	1.42
6	Schools, Medical	37	3.09	3.77	22	Research	9	0.75	5.36
7	Teaching	31	2.59	2.01	23	Computer-Assisted Instruction	9	0.75	1.67
8	Clinical Competence	24	2.01	1.05					
9	Faculty, Medical	23	1.92	0.63	24	Interviews as Topic	8	0.67	9.57
10	Clinical Clerkship	23	1.92	4.27	25	Staff Development	7	0.59	3.93
11	Pediatrics	22	1.84	1.55	26	Physicians	7	0.59	0.40
12	Internal Medicine	19	1.59	1.85	27	Patient-Centered Care	7	0.59	4.21
13	Problem-Based Learning	18	1.51	3.15	28	Medical Staff, Hospital	7	0.59	1.48
14	Education, Medical, Graduate	16	1.34	0.34	29	Burnout, Professional	7	0.59	1.59
15	Stress, Psychological	15	1.25	5.21	30	Social Media	7	0.59	7.38

Figure 52　Highest frequent MeSH terms of *Medical Education Online*

7. *Journal of Surgical Education* (Figure 53)

Ranking	MeSH Term	Frequency	Percentage (A)	A/O	Ranking	MeSH Term	Frequency	Percentage (A)	A/O
1	General Surgery	762	17.48	8.57	16	Orthopedic Procedures	32	0.73	4.87
2	Education, Medical, Graduate	342	7.84	1.96	17	Faculty, Medical	32	0.73	1.00
3	Internship and Residency	323	7.41	1.47	18	Competency-Based Education	31	0.71	2.03
					19	Urology	30	0.69	1.86
4	Laparoscopy	129	2.96	4.70	20	Personnel Selection	29	0.67	3.19
5	Education, Medical, Undergraduate	116	2.66	0.80	21	Cholecystectomy, Laparoscopic	28	0.64	8.00
6	Simulation Training	101	2.32	58.00	22	Teaching	28	0.64	0.50
7	Specialties, Surgical	98	2.25	6.25	23	Biomedical Research	27	0.62	0.98
8	Orthopedics	94	2.16	3.84	24	Workload	27	0.62	2.70
9	Educational Measurement	68	1.56	0.88	25	Clinical Competence	27	0.62	0.32
10	Students, Medical	54	1.24	0.35	26	Gynecology	27	0.62	1.38
11	Surgery, Plastic	40	0.92	2.79	27	Patient Care Team	26	0.60	2.22
12	Surgeons	39	0.89	1.78	28	Vascular Surgical Procedures	26	0.60	3.16
13	Suture Techniques	38	0.87	7.25	29	Traumatology	26	0.60	4.62
14	Clinical Clerkship	34	0.78	1.73	30	Robotic Surgical Procedures	25	0.57	3.35
15	Education, Medical	33	0.76	0.16					

Figure 53　Highest frequent MeSH terms of *Journal of Surgical Education*

8. *BMC Medical Education* (Figure 54)

Ranking	MeSH Term	Frequency	Percentage (A)	A/O	Ranking	MeSH Term	Frequency	Percentage (A)	A/O
1	Students, Medical	551	9.64	2.69	16	General Practice	52	0.91	2.07
2	Education, Medical, Undergraduate	314	5.50	1.65	17	Stress, Psychological	45	0.79	3.29
					18	Pediatrics	45	0.79	0.66
3	Clinical Competence	256	4.48	2.35	19	Education, Medical, Continuing	44	0.77	0.46
4	Education, Medical	175	3.06	0.65	20	Health Occupations	42	0.74	3.70
5	Educational Measurement	160	2.80	1.65	21	Students, Health Occupations	42	0.74	6.73
6	Internship and Residency	116	2.03	0.40	22	Biomedical Research	42	0.74	1.17
7	Problem-Based Learning	93	1.63	3.40	23	Computer-Assisted Instruction	41	0.72	1.60
8	Education, Medical, Graduate	91	1.59	0.40	24	Students, Nursing	38	0.67	7.44
9	Teaching	86	1.51	1.17	25	Physical Therapy Specialty	36	0.63	10.50
10	Physicians	79	1.38	0.94	26	Professional Competence	34	0.60	3.75
11	Health Personnel	72	1.26	2.38	27	Clinical Clerkship	33	0.58	1.29
12	Schools, Medical	64	1.12	1.37	28	Evidence-Based Medicine	32	0.56	2.80
13	Internal Medicine	60	1.05	1.22					
14	Faculty, Medical	55	0.96	1.32	29	Family Practice	32	0.56	0.75
15	Medical Staff, Hospital	53	0.93	2.33	30	Burnout, Professional	32	0.56	1.51

Figure 54   Highest frequent MeSH terms of *BMC Medical Education*

9. *Teaching and Learning in Medicine* (Figure 55)

Ranking	MeSH Term	Frequency	Percentage (A)	A/O	Ranking	MeSH Term	Frequency	Percentage (A)	A/O
1	Students, Medical	130	13.61	3.79	16	Curriculum	12	1.26	1.75
2	Education, Medical, Undergraduate	77	8.06	2.41	17	Emergency Medicine	11	1.15	1.28
					18	Physical Examination	10	1.08	7.71
3	Educational Measurement	52	5.45	3.21	19	General Surgery	9	0.94	0.46
4	Clinical Competence	43	4.50	2.36	20	Physicians	9	0.94	0.64
5	Teaching	40	4.19	3.25	21	Preceptorship	9	0.94	11.75
6	Education, Medical	34	3.56	0.76	22	Staff Development	8	0.84	5.60
7	Internal Medicine	31	3.25	3.78	23	Health Personnel	8	0.84	1.58
8	Education, Medical, Graduate	25	2.62	0.66	24	Problem-Based Learning	7	0.73	1.52
9	Pediatrics	20	2.09	0.84	25	Stress, Psychological	7	0.73	3.04
10	Clinical Clerkship	20	2.09	4.64	26	Surveys and Questionnaires	6	0.63	7.88
11	Faculty, Medical	19	1.99	2.73	27	Professional Competence	6	0.63	3.94
12	Internship and Residency	18	1.88	0.17	28	Anatomy	5	0.52	0.66
13	Schools, Medical	15	1.57	1.91	29	Obstetrics	5	0.52	0.18
14	Competency-Based Education	13	1.36	3.89	30	Biomedical Research	5	0.52	0.83
15	Family Practice	12	1.26	1.68					

Figure 55   Highest frequent MeSH terms of *Teaching and Learning in Medicine*

10. *Academic Psychiatry* (Figure 56)

Ranking	MeSH Term	Frequency	Percentage (A)	A/O	Ranking	MeSH Term	Frequency	Percentage (A)	A/O
1	Psychiatry	786	22.63	22.86	16	Psychotherapy	38	1.09	12.11
2	Internship and Residency	252	7.25	1.44	17	Educational Measurement	38	1.09	0.64
3	Students, Medical	194	5.58	1.55	18	Suicide	35	1.01	16.83
4	Curriculum	80	2.30	3.19	19	Stress, Psychological	32	0.92	3.83
5	Physicians	73	2.10	1.43	20	Mental Health Services	30	0.86	21.50
6	Mental Disorders	64	1.84	12.27	21	Depression	29	0.83	6.92
7	Education, Medical, Graduate	58	1.67	0.42	22	Biomedical Research	28	0.81	1.29
					23	Teaching	23	0.66	0.51
8	Child Psychiatry	50	1.44	24.00	24	Schools, Medical	22	0.63	0.77
9	Education, Medical	49	1.41	0.30	25	Substance-Related Disorders	22	0.63	7.88
10	Clinical Competence	47	1.35	0.71					
11	Clinical Clerkship	46	1.32	2.93	26	Neurosciences	19	0.55	13.75
12	Burnout, Professional	43	1.24	3.35	27	Fellowships and Scholarships	17	0.49	1.53
13	Education, Medical, Undergraduate	41	1.18	0.35	28	Academic Medical Centers	15	0.43	1.59
14	Adolescent Psychiatry	39	1.12	22.50	29	Forensic Psychiatry	15	0.43	21.50
15	Faculty, Medical	38	1.09	1.49	30	Cultural Competency	14	0.40	4.00

Figure 56   Highest frequent MeSH terms of *Academic Psychiatry*

Conclusions

The year 2022 marks the fifth annual release of the International Medical Education Research Fronts Report. The distinction of this current volume can be found in its thorough review and comparison of medical education research hotspots and developments over the last two decades as well as the introduction of an additional special series on teaching in medical education at a global level. Through literature overview and tracking of research fronts, we can keep up with the pace of medical education development and promote exchanges, cooperation, research and innovation in countries all over the world.